STOP WORRYING

ABOUT YOUR HEALTH!

How to Quit
Obsessing About Symptoms
and Feel Better Now

George D. Zgourides, M.D., Psy.D.

Lulu Press

Edited by Heather Mitchener
Text design by Tracy Powell-Carlson

ISBN: 978-1-4357-1192-1

To Dad

Contents

Introduction

Illness is not something a person *has*. It's another way
of being.

—Jonathan Miller

As a clinical psychologist, I encounter many patients who suffer from health anxiety. Some manage to function fairly well; others do not. What all of these people have in common is a preoccupation with health that affects their lives in diverse ways. Consider the following cases:

> Doris is a thirty-six-year-old woman with a history of frequent doctor visits and medical tests. Prior to beginning psychotherapy, Doris had lost her younger sister (age thirty- two) to a baffling illness involving both lupus and multiple sclerosis (MS). Understandably, Doris reported a few months of severe depression and distress over her sister's death. Then, without warning, she also began experiencing some symptoms identical to those her sister had had before dying.
>
> This caused Doris to fall into an even deeper depression, mainly over fears that she, too, was going to die a painful death at any time. Doris spent time "doctor shopping," looking for a physician who could offer her both an official diagnosis and some words of comfort. But medical tests never showed anything wrong. Her symptoms seemed to mimic lupus and MS, yet successive exams and lab tests couldn't confirm a disease. Quite often, Doris was told to see another physician and have another exotic test. In some instances, she was given a prescription for antidepressants, or even condescendingly told "there's nothing we can do for you" and dismissed with a pat on the back. Still, Doris had a nagging feeling that something must be amiss, which, in her mind, also meant something could be done to alleviate her symptoms and worries.
>
> A cousin suggested that Doris try counseling. Doris was absolutely *livid* that anyone would imply that her problems were "all in her head," and she adamantly refused to go. Meanwhile, whenever Doris thought about her sister or felt stressed, her symptoms would become much worse. And she'd worry even more about being sick.
>
> After losing countless nights of sleep and finding no answers to her complaints, Doris finally took her cousin's advice and made an appointment with me.
>
> Within several sessions, Doris began to show some improvement in her health-related anxieties as she learned to modify her irrational thinking patterns. She also came to realize how the stresses of her sister's death, and the emotional conflicts over losing so close a family member,

had contributed to her developing bodily symptoms as well as an incessant worry over having a deadly disease. At the same time, Doris made several important lifestyle changes: daily writing in a journal, learning yoga, exercising three times a week, and controlling her intake of sugar and caffeine. As she slowly developed a more realistic and accepting attitude about her own life (and inevitable death), her uncomfortable symptoms and disease anxieties began to diminish.

And another patient's story:

Eric, a twenty-one-year-old college student, was admitted late one night to a hospital with complaints of a choking sensation. His college roommates brought him to the local emergency room, where they told the attending physician about Eric's episode.

While Eric had always shown a tendency toward being "a hypochondriac" (their words), his health worries had worsened in recent weeks. Although perfectly normal in every other way, Eric had long complained about headaches, backaches, and stomach problems. He was also known to frequent the student health center looking for "something that'll work this time" (Eric's words).

Eric was planning a career in nursing, but the further along he advanced in his schooling, the more stressful life became for him. He was having extra trouble in his senior nursing courses, as well as becoming panicky about upcoming board exams he needed to pass in order to practice as a nurse.

During the week prior to his emergency room visit, Eric had slept little due to a great deal of late-night studying for finals. His roommates all agreed that Eric had been under exceptional stress when he suddenly started to feel that he was choking. Upon arriving at the hospital, Eric was examined and given numerous tests. When the doctors found nothing physically wrong with him, they did their best to reassure him and to persuade him to lighten up on the stressors in his life. Later that night, Eric was discharged and sent back to his dorm room with a prescription for a minor tranquilizer.

Soon after this episode at the hospital, and at the urging of his friends and the staff of the college health center, Eric agreed to schedule an appointment with me.

In therapy, he has shown improvement in his understanding of his health-related anxieties.

As you can see from their stories, people like Doris and Eric worry about their health. Most are hyperaware of their bodies, discerning and fretting over bodily sensations that most people don't even notice. Some might focus on health-related matters, have multiple lab tests, and never quite believe they aren't deathly ill. Others might be sure they have a particular disease, but be too frightened to see a health-care practitioner. Some will read about one disease and obsess over it. Others will manage to acquire a "disease of the week," as their symptoms mysteriously move from one part of the body to another. Whatever the manifestation, these people share a common clinical feature: *anxiety over their health*.

Most of us have felt the need to scratch when a friend shows us his new rash. Indeed, at one time or another, almost all of us experience uncomfortable physical sensations that cause us some concern or doubt.

But this type of sporadic health worry isn't what I mean by *health anxiety*—I'm referring to the phenomenon of feeling *overcome* by your health worries to the point where they cause distress or even interfere with your daily activities and relationships. It's one thing to have an occasional minor headache or a cold. It's another thing to worry about getting a headache or cold, or to think you have something worse, like a brain hemorrhage or tuberculosis.

You may worry excessively that you're ill—even after doctors have assured you you're not and medical tests have confirmed these assurances. Or you may suffer from a milder preoccupation with your health that can interfere with enjoying the health you have. You might develop health anxieties for short periods of time—less than six months—after a friend is afflicted with a disease or you learn that someone in your family is ill. You're normal in every other respect; you work, go to school, and socialize. You don't have a mental disorder; you just worry too much about your health.

As a clinical psychologist with expertise in anxiety disorders and mind-body psychology (also called health psychology), I want to help you understand your preoccupation with physical illness and symptoms and learn how to counter these through the use of some basic self-help psychological strategies. You'll learn how to identify your own causes of excessive worry, counteract irrational self-talk about minor, everyday physical symptoms, and finally accept and redefine your experience of your symptoms.

In the following pages, I'll describe the phenomenon of *health anxiety syndrome*, a term I've coined to refer to what is popularly known as health anxiety, health obsession, or disease phobia. Even though there are some gradations in meaning across this nomenclature, I'll use these terms interchangeably and somewhat loosely throughout this book. For example, when I refer to a disease phobic, I'm talking about someone who worries about catching diseases, and not someone who has a diagnosable phobic disorder.

Practical Pointer

Health anxiety syndrome is a general descriptor for the condition affecting individuals who worry too much about their health.

What Is Health Anxiety Syndrome?

All of us endure minor ailments, and most of us ignore them. However, for people with health anxiety syndrome, even little symptoms take on larger-than-life meaning. A headache following a long day at work means a brain tumor. Soreness after exercise spells leukemia. A racing heart following an exciting movie means heart disease. A new freckle on the skin translates into melanoma.

Making matters worse, the worry can become so great that new symptoms arise in response to the anxiety (for example, panic attacks, insomnia, tightness in the chest, etc.). Disease phobics are also prone to developing new fears and symptoms from what they've recently seen or read in the media (e.g., reports on increasing numbers of outbreaks of mad cow disease and anthrax), after witnessing a health trauma (e.g., a bloody accident), or after learning about a loved one's physical problems. Symptoms can also be exacerbated by general life stressors.

Here's how one patient described his health worries:

> It's a major hassle, and I know it's irrational. But I can't help it. For heaven's sake, I break out into cold sweats when the news mentions the latest outbreak of some disease like ebola in Africa.

And another client described her anxiety:

I'll lose sleep over the thought of not being to obtain this year's flu shot. What if I can't get one? What if I catch a terrible flu? Then I worry about dying prematurely from some flesh-devouring disease.

Does any of this sound familiar? If you experience health anxiety syndrome, you perpetually fret about your body. The slightest sensation makes you worry that you're going to have to undergo surgery, take nausea-causing medications, or die prematurely. And going to the doctor doesn't help. Nor do lab tests that say you're okay. Everyone tells you that you're fine, but you can't believe them. You just know in your heart that something is wrong. Very wrong.

Your anxiety seems to have taken on a life of its own. And if your preoccupation is severe enough, it can be damaging to all the parts of your life: family, work, home, and school. Just think back on how your health worries have interrupted your lifestyle.

This problem is more complicated than a mere label might suggest. Commonly, health anxieties first involve minor physical symptoms (an intermittent cough, a skin rash), bodily processes (sweating, breathing, digestion, and elimination), vague sensations (nonspecific pain, fatigue, numbness), or a combination of these that specifically catch your attention. Rather than shrugging off the sensations as a normal aggravation, you then attribute your symptoms to a particular disease, though you won't get a diagnosis from medical professionals. Why? Because, as you'll learn in this book, what you have is not an actual disease. But neither can health anxiety be dismissed outright as an imagined problem, although many non-sufferers will try to do that. Unfortunately, uncertainty becomes a way of life. You're never quite sure if a symptom like sore muscles is a simple nuisance or if you're truly ill with a condition like multiple sclerosis.

Millions of Americans suffer from health anxieties of one sort or another. Ranging in severity from minor to intense, this syndrome affects men and women of all ages, races, ethnic backgrounds, sexual orientations, and religions. People who have health anxieties come from all walks of life, including white-collar professionals, blue-collar workers, teachers, attorneys, artists, medical professionals, engineers, and so on.

Yet, little information on health anxiety is published for average readers. Nor is compassion a common reaction of the general public or medical professionals. Unfortunately, because of this dearth of information and all-too-common insensitivity directed at those with health anxiety, few resources are available for sufferers or those who care for them. This observation, in part, originally inspired me to write *Stop Worrying About Your Health!*

Trouble for All

In its more severe manifestations, health anxiety disrupts the lives of sufferers and places pressure on those closest to them—spouses, children, parents, friends, coworkers, bosses, and health-care practitioners. The emotional pain associated with this problem can be severe and incapacitating. From the mother who is unable to take her children to the park for fear of catching germs, to the father who refuses to eat any fat for fear of having a heart attack, to the college student who overexercises to keep in shape, to the teenager who can't sleep for fear of having an incurable disease, to the woman who misses too much work for repeated medical appointments, health anxiety syndrome can exert a damaging effect on lives.

A case in point: I was rather surprised when an attorney friend of mine called to tell me she couldn't stop worrying about "catching HIV" from breathing the same air as an infected person. For the past six months, she had worried about being in the same room as someone who was coughing or sneezing. No matter how much I tried to reassure my friend that HIV isn't transmitted through the air, she took little comfort in my words. Her legal practice was suffering, so she finally sought psychological help. Her case underscores the reality that people of any age, background, and occupation can have health anxieties.

The effects on families can be exhausting. Frequent medical appointments. Filling out new paperwork for each new doctor. Listening to continual griping about health problems. Making late-night trips to the emergency room. Never being able to make plans that involve being very far from a hospital. It's enough to wear out even the most forgiving of us.

To complicate matters, significant others rarely have a place to turn to express their concerns or process their feelings about trying to live with someone who has excessive health worries. Resentment and hurt feelings can also build over the years, to such a degree that marriages and other relationships are strained. Moreover, health anxiety syndrome can occasionally function as a coping mechanism—or *secondary gain*—that relieves sufferers of some responsibility (for example, "I'm sick, so I can't cut the grass today"). Secondary gain refers to your reactions that assist in sustaining your problems, usually by reinforcing them. In other words, you receive some indirect reward from staying sick. Examples include attention from the family, financial incentives, and avoidance of undesirable situations. This is in contrast to *primary gain*, in which your problems directly satisfy some psychological need or conflict. In other words, your problems serve an important psychological purpose and resolve a conflict that you might not otherwise be able to handle. Both secondary and primary gains can be present in health anxiety syndrome and cause a good deal of stress for significant others.

The strain of health anxiety on our nation's medical system is another problem. Excessive and time-consuming office appointments, physical exams, emergency room visits, phone calls for reassurance, surgeries, and medical tests—including blood and urine lab work, X-rays, multiple resonance imaging (MRIs), and computerized axial tomography (CAT scans)—are costly. And, ironically, complications from excessive use of the above (such as injury from multiple X-rays) is a real possibility. In this way, excessive heath concerns become a self-fulfilling prophecy; your fears lead to behaviors that lead to consequences that fulfill your original fears. Health anxiety syndrome is an expensive problem in more ways than one—you and others pay financially, emotionally, and physically.

Even in its less severe—and perhaps much more common—manifestations, health anxiety is a downright nuisance. It interferes with your ability to enjoy life. Your worries might not disrupt your job or your marriage, but you don't enjoy life like you previously did. You'd like not to have any fears about your health. You'd like to pick up a magazine and not immediately think you have the latest disease that's described in an article. You'd like not to notice a long list of everyday aches and pains. You'd like to get a good night's sleep and feel refreshed in the morning. *You want to feel normal again.*

Practical Pointer

In its more severe forms, health anxiety syndrome disrupts the lives of sufferers and places pressure on those closest to them: spouses, children, parents, friends, coworkers, bosses, and health-care practitioners. In its less severe forms, health anxiety syndrome causes distress and interferes with a person's ability to enjoy life.

Avoiding Psychological Help: A Real Enigma

Health anxiety syndrome is a deep mystery to its sufferers; you have no idea why you feel so bad and worry so much about your health—you just do. This might make you demand special consideration and treatment from those around you, as well as refuse to discuss your problem with the one type of doctor who might be able help you: a psychologist or psychiatrist. You instead find it easier to "doctor shop" and pay for medical tests in the hopes of identifying a "real" illness. Unfortunately, no amount of medical treatment or professional solace helps to allay your fears of disease and germs. You resist referrals to mental health clinicians, and frustration and anger are frequent on both sides of the doctor's desk.

Clearly, at least when major symptoms arise, it's wise to check with a health-care professional to rule out an actual disease state. After a second or third opinion confirms a lack of any findings, it's time for you to consider the possibility that a psychological process is generating your symptoms—a phenomenon known as *somatization*, which we'll explore in chapter 1.

Once you realize nothing is actually wrong with you physically (after you've had a multitude of medical appointments and tests, all of which turn up nothing), you might experience serious embarrassment over your health fears. You might think you've made a fool of yourself in front of your physicians, family, and acquaintances. You might feel guilty and ashamed. You might become very angry. Or you might isolate yourself with the mistaken belief that no one else has this problem or truly understands your plight.

Please know that *you're not alone!* You don't need to feel foolish or embarrassed or angry. But you do need to face up to the fact that you're your own worst enemy when it comes to your health anxieties.

What Causes It?

And the cause of health anxieties? Like the cause of all forms of anxiety, no one knows for sure, but experts suspect a combination of factors.

Health anxieties probably arise in response to both a genetic predisposition to nervousness and various life experience "triggers," although scientists aren't certain how this process occurs exactly.

What is suspected is that a history of childhood illnesses plays a part in the eventual emergence of health anxiety syndrome, which is often directly preceded by a major life event or trauma. This triggering event can be a onetime occurrence (for example, the death of a parent) or a continual occurrence (severe work-related stress). Once activated, though, health anxieties are reinforced through sympathy or attention (whether positive or negative) from family members, friends, neighbors, and the health-care system. Over time, the preoccupation with bodily symptoms becomes a part of everyday life.

From a slightly different angle, life stressors, whether severe or not, can alter your general attitude and mood. The same is true of unresolved psychological conflicts—those emotional needs and upsets that we all have deep inside but haven't worked through. In fact, your unresolved conflicts can directly cause your physical symptoms, which then cause you to worry.

Thus, any change in your psychological perceptions and interpretations of events can trigger bodily ailments, ranging from skin rashes to back pain to migraines, that are related to the initial stress. You then convince yourself that you're infected with some sort of pathogen, or even worse, that you've developed a life-threatening disease like cancer. This triggers more stress. You go to doctor after doctor, only to be disappointed at hearing nothing is wrong, which triggers even more stress. And if you receive any attention or special consideration for your symptoms, this will also tend to reinforce the idea of your having health problems.

Practical Pointer

For reasons not fully understood, stress and unresolved psychological conflicts can manifest as physical symptoms, including excessive worry about those symptoms. When this happens, a vicious cycle of stress, symptoms, more stress, medical worries, and even more stress begins and continues until interrupted.

Is There Hope?

You've probably noticed that family and doctors tend to dismiss your health anxieties as "imagined" or "feigned." But ignoring health anxiety syndrome isn't likely to do much good. Let's face it, if the problem were going to go away on its own, it would've done so already, right?

Rest assured, there is good news—self-help psychological treatment for your health anxieties is possible. And it works. Because the primary culprit in health anxiety syndrome is your thought processes, the cure lies within the realm of your mind. In other words, the primary method used to overcome this problem is learning to rethink your life experiences and interpretations of physical symptoms and complaints. Such *cognitive reframing*, which I'll explain in detail in later chapters, is easily accomplished within a self-help format. This means you can enjoy complete control of your own therapy, which should also reduce the inherent stress and shame associated with facing your problem and embracing the methods that can help you overcome your worries.

Practical Pointer

Because the primary culprit in health anxiety syndrome is your thought processes, the cure lies within the realm of rethinking your life experiences and interpretations of physical symptoms and complaints.

Stop Worrying About Your Health! contains seven chapters that offer you important information on this troublesome problem. Topics addressed include what health anxiety syndrome is and how to determine if you or someone else has it; what mind-body psychology is and how it's related to health anxiety; the causes of excessive health worries; cognitive-behavioral self-help methods and other psychological and medical treatments; the role of family, social support, and complementary health approaches; and various personal accounts from sufferers.

I'm sure you'll agree that public awareness of and education in regard to health anxiety syndrome are needed, and it's my hope this book will play a part in bringing this about.

Health anxiety syndrome can be an uncomfortable problem, but it doesn't have to be. Readied with the information and techniques presented in the following pages, you can overcome it and regain control of your life. May the information and resources contained in *Stop Worrying About Your Health!* help you to find freedom from all of your health anxieties.

Feature: Why Self-Help Therapy?

As a clinical psychologist, I'm often asked why I'm such a strong proponent of self-help therapy. I think of self-help therapy as *deliberate self-coping*. And that's why I've written *Stop Worrying About Your Health!* I want you to have the tools necessary to help yourself overcome your health anxieties.

You can learn to handle your own distressing situations by exercising intentional conscious control. You can learn to change your own thoughts, feelings, and behaviors. You can learn to recognize your own personal flaws and decide to master your circumstances and your life. Perhaps nothing in life is as empowering as knowing you can take control and work to solve your own problems.

This isn't to say you have to go it alone. Whenever possible, you should seek support from your significant others and family members. And there are times when you should seek professional help; there's nothing shameful about that. But, in many instances, you can learn to help yourself without the expense of seeing a psychologist or other health-care professional. Self-help therapy, then, becomes *self-improvement, self-responsibility*, and *self-reliance*.

If the idea of helping yourself overcome health anxiety syndrome seems a little unrealistic, then remember that our society encourages us to be changed by others rather than change ourselves. If the idea of self-help therapy makes sense to you—and I hope it does—then you obviously understand that every time you make plans, imagine a better way, weigh alternatives, or solve problems, you're engaging in self-helping behavior.

I imagine many of us don't think about all of the opportunities we have to improve our lives. Instead, we feel controlled by others, circumstances, or whatever. Or we feel powerless to problem-solve or develop our coping skills.

A peaceful and prosperous life, while requiring lots of motivation and hard work on your part, is within your grasp—if you'll only take the challenge to think about your life in a new way.

Before you move on to chapter 1, give some thought to your goals for reading *Stop Worrying About Your Health!*

1

Do You Have Health Anxiety Syndrome?

If you mean to keep as well as possible, the less you think about your health the better.

—Oliver Wendell Holmes, Sr.

Take a moment and reflect on these comments from several of my clients:

> *I just can't help it. I worry a lot about catching some germ. Any little thing that goes wrong with my body, I think it's cancer or another deadly disease. I realize I'm being completely illogical, but I still worry.*

> *I'm tired of going from doctor to doctor, as well as never getting an answer as to why I'm always catching colds.*

> *The medical tests always come up negative. They tell me I'm in great shape for a thirty-two-year-old, even though I'm sure I've got a terminal illness.*

> *I exercise constantly, because I'm anxious all the time about losing my good health and good looks.*

> *Hardly a minute of the day goes by when I'm not thinking about what hurts, what might be wrong, or if I'm going to die.*

> *If I think about my back pain for too long, I can convince myself that I've got malignant tumors in my lower spine. Some nights I can't sleep from worrying; I'll even start crying over all this nonsense.*

Have you ever tossed and turned in bed for hours, worrying that you have a dreaded disease? Have you ever gone from one doctor to another, only to have them assure you there's absolutely nothing wrong? Are you plagued by such symptoms as headaches, back pain, tingling, numbness, heart palpitations, excess stomach acid, alternating diarrhea and constipation, muscle spasms, eye twitches, rashes, fear of going crazy, fear of looking foolish, or fear of dying? Because of your symptoms, are you anxious about having cancer, heart disease, multiple sclerosis, HIV, or any other severe disorder? Have you ever felt as if your body gets in the way of your marriage, family, friends, job, school, or any other aspect of your life?

If you're bothered by any of the above, know that you have plenty of company! Literally millions of Americans experience the same problem you do: health anxiety.

Over the years, I've worked with many people with health anxieties—so many that I started conceptualizing a general syndrome that includes excessive worries about bodily sensations that, for one reason or another, don't truly qualify for a full-fledged diagnosis. In other words, a lot of everyday Americans are preoccupied by health matters, and it bothers them and disrupts life to some extent. But they don't actually have a mental disorder like obsessive-compulsive disorder, or hypochondria, or a phobia. Yes, they have tendencies that resemble these, but not the actual disorders. (In clinical psychology, this phenomenon is referred to as "subclinical.") This and many other observations—especially the one that anyone with health worries is categorically (and insultingly) labeled a "hypochondriac"—led me to write this book.

What Is Health Anxiety Syndrome?

Briefly, health anxiety syndrome refers to *undue worry about your health*. The anxiety can range from occasional and mild worry to more chronic and intense anxiety. Depending on your unique experience of health anxiety, you might suffer from one or more of the following:

- Nervousness at the thought of having health problems

- Hypersensitivity (being overly alert) to bodily symptoms

- Overreaction to bodily symptoms

- Obsessive thinking about health, illness, germs, dirt, etc.

- Compulsive behaviors, like refusing to touch certain objects (such as toilet seats)

- A tendency to overinterpret (catastrophize about) symptoms, such as thinking a bruise *will* turn into a deadly blood clot

- A tendency to exaggerate everyday symptoms

- A tendency to seek multiple medical opinions in hope of finding a "real" answer

- A tendency to worry excessively about diet, fat, and getting enough exercise

- A tendency to use physical complaints and symptoms to receive attention and comfort or to find freedom from responsibility (secondary gain)

Or as another one of my patients described his experience of disease anxiety:

> I've had health anxieties, maybe hypochondria, for most
> of my adult life. It's hard to admit this, but it's the truth.
> My problem seems to be under control, maybe because
> I'm on antidepressants. Most of the people I know don't
> realize that mine is an actual problem. They seem to get
> the idea that fear can't overwhelm you. Before I went into
> counseling, my life was pretty difficult because I couldn't
> seem to stop thinking or talking about my ailments. Even
> today, on a really bad day, I'm convinced I have one or
> more serious diseases like AIDS and muscular dystrophy.
> Doctors will tell me one thing, but my body tells me
> something entirely different. This problem is probably a
> lot like obsessive-compulsive disorder, at least what I know
> about it.

Having health anxiety syndrome, in whatever form and to whatever degree, means being overly alert to your body and worrying about health problems, anything ranging from a chronic, annoying nuisance condition (for example, seasonal allergies) to a serious, even terminal one (such as brain cancer). The point here is that it's not the seriousness of the perceived illness that counts, it's the fact you're hypersensitive to sensations in your body, which in turn lays the groundwork for you to worry about having a health condition.

If you experience health anxiety syndrome, you might also have many of the same signs as people with anxiety disorders: nervousness, pounding heart, panic, muscle tension, tingling or numbness in the limbs, changes in eating patterns, changes in sleeping patterns, headaches, and muscle tension. There are a couple of differences, though: your anxiety centers around your physical symptoms and health, and it falls short of being fully diagnosable.

The realization that what appears to be unreasonable behavior is actually an honest expression of inner turmoil—and that others have the same experience—can be a source of relief. In this way, the battle against health anxieties becomes, not a fight against shadows or illusions, but a fight against an identifiable problem. It's at this point that many disease phobics will decide to seek professional help for their health anxieties instead of for their bodily symptoms, often at the urging of their significant others. Armed with information, support, and understanding from family and friends, seeking help becomes a less intimidating task.

And this makes practical sense. After all, you don't want to be ill. In fact, you'd be thrilled to feel utterly confident that you're fine. You could get a full night's sleep if only you knew in your soul that nothing is physically wrong. No one wants to have health anxiety. It's frightening.

Practical Pointer

Experiencing health anxiety syndrome means being afraid you have a condition or disease, anything from a chronic nuisance problem to a serious, even terminal one. It's not the seriousness of the perceived illness that determines if you experience health anxiety syndrome, it's that 1) you're overly sensitive to sensations in your body and 2) you worry about having a health condition.

Not a Diagnosis

During my years in clinical practice, I've treated many people with health worries that easily qualify for one of the usual diagnostic categories, like hypochondria. Their symptoms nicely fit the published criteria. Their problem is unmistakable, so their answer is unmistakable. They proceed with treatment without excessive difficulty.

But life isn't always so straightforward. I've also treated many people who don't qualify for one of the usual categories. Their symptoms just don't match the expected criteria. And while maybe not severe enough to warrant an official diagnosis as defined by the American Psychiatric Association, their complaints are bothersome enough to warrant reading a self-help book or coming to me for short-term counseling.

We live in a medicalized society that wants to label all uncomfortable emotional problems as bona fide mental disorders. Doing this seems to lessen people's guilt or shame at having psychological issues. After all, if it's diagnosable, then it's somehow legitimate. And that means there must be a quick-fix answer out there somewhere, if only the right specialist can be found.

However, I take the opposite approach and resist applying diagnostic labels in all cases where people worry about their health. In other words, I, like any ethical clinician, avoid using diagnostic labels unless I think there's a good reason for doing so—such as when my patients meet established criteria. Health anxiety syndrome is not a diagnosis—it's a general way of describing the broader phenomenon of health-related worries.

Even though our society relies on labels to a certain extent, the flip side is that those labels can result in social stigmas. As one example, having OCD (obsessive-compulsive disorder) usually carries with it images of sufferers bleaching down the entire house, ironing bed sheets, and washing their hands hundreds of times each day to avoid contaminants. While this might be true of some actual OCD sufferers, it's not true of everyone who worries about their health, frets about touching soiled objects or catching germs, or refuses to use public toilet seats. In other words, you can have uncomfortable thoughts about diseases and germs without necessarily qualifying for a psychiatric diagnosis of OCD. See how this works?

As another example, consider the social stigmas related to the label "psychosomatic," which implies having physical problems that aren't real, which further implies "it's all in your head." This isn't the case. If it were, you wouldn't feel any physical symptoms. A psychosomatic problem might be generated in your psyche, but it's experienced in your body. The mind-body connection, which we'll explore in the next chapter, simply can't be ignored. Nonetheless, being seen as having a psychosomatic problem can leave people feeling as if they're "neurotics" with ridiculous symptoms who should stop acting so crazily and quit bothering their doctors.

The problem of labeling also extends to hypochondria. Calling someone a "hypochondriac" can be tantamount to an insult. The implication is that these are pitiable and lonely individuals who love to talk only about their sicknesses. As so aptly described by Carla Cantor (1996) in her book, *Phantom Illness: Recognizing, Understanding, and Overcoming Hypochondria*:

> Doctors typically treat hypochondriacs with disrespect. Derogatorily referred to as "crocks," hypochondriacs are thought to be self-centered complainers who believe they are ill when they are not and who reject all help that doctors try to provide. Doctors find it frustrating to provide the repeated reassurance these patients crave, and many do not consider them to be truly troubled or medically ill. (p. ix)

Hence, with the exception of cases in which a true mental illness is present (and I might still argue against certain practices of modern diagnostic labeling), I don't see how applying what amounts for some people to be belittling name-calling is of any benefit to anyone.

Not surprisingly, those of you who experience health anxiety syndrome, as a group, don't exactly welcome the idea of being given a psychological label. You probably see any hint that you might have an emotional issue as asinine and insulting. In your mind, having a psychological condition is perhaps identical to having a moral defect or personal weakness. While completely untrue, our society fosters such nonsense. If you're moral and strong, you're supposed to be able to solve your own problems. Such irrationality can become the source of your "blind spot"—denial of the role that psychological factors play in your difficulties. You might reject needed counseling, and instead continue to seek more and more medical treatments, which of course prove useless, costly, and time-consuming for all.

As I'll show in upcoming chapters, you don't have to believe what other people tell you about illness or disease-related worries. You're not immoral, weak, or villainous in any way because you have health anxieties.

Practical Pointer

You don't have to believe what other people tell you about illness or health worries. You're not immoral, weak, or villainous in any way because you have health anxieties.

For now, though, keep in mind that having "subclinical" health worries doesn't mean having a diagnosable mental disorder. Yes, many millions of Americans suffer from full-blown mental disorders. And for these folks, a number of psychological and medical treatments are available from licensed health-care professionals. But millions of you fall short of a diagnosable disorder; you don't have a mental illness. Instead, you worry excessively about your health, and this bothers you. You might even have *characteristics* that resemble particular disorders, like obsessive-compulsive disorder or hypochondria. But you're basically fine, with the exception of your excessive health worries. It's especially for you that I've written this self-help book.

Let me repeat, *health anxiety syndrome isn't a diagnosis.* It's a general way of describing the broader phenomenon of health-related worries.

Practical Pointer

Millions of you have health anxieties that fall short of a diagnosable disorder. You're basically fine, except you worry too much about your health, and this bothers you.

What's Going On?

You might be wondering, "If I don't have a mental disorder, what's causing my health anxieties?" No one knows for certain what mental processes underlie excessive health worries. However, psychologists do implicate two different, but related, processes in the experience of health worries. One process involves *somatization*; the other involves *anxiousness*. I'll describe them both below.

Regardless of your unique experiences with health anxiety, you can overcome your health worries and move on with your life. The first step, however, is understanding what your problem is. So, let's take a quick look at these two basic psychological processes involved in health anxiety syndrome.

Practical Pointer

If you experience health anxiety syndrome—a broad descriptor for chronic health worries—you don't necessarily have a full-blown mental disorder. You may instead have characteristics that resemble one or more mental disorders without all of the usual clinical features.

Somatization

Somatization is the process whereby you develop physical symptoms in response to psychological issues, often with an accompanying pre-occupation with, and overreporting of, bodily sensations. You're conscious of a multitude of physical symptoms—many seemingly unrelated—that seem to rule your life, but you're not conscious of the mental conflicts that are producing your symptoms. Obviously, many cases of health anxiety syndrome involve some element of somatization.

The causes of somatization continue to elude researchers. Robert Kellner (1991), in his book, *Psychosomatic Syndrome and Somatic Symptoms*, presented his theories on the development of somatoform symptoms in patients:

> One person may have distressing somatic symptoms because of physiological disturbances with genetic factors predisposing, whereas another may have somatic symptoms only when he or she is anxious or depressed. Another may attend to somatic symptoms only when she fears that she has a disease, whereas another may habitually attend to bodily sensations because of early learning. Yet another may complain of bodily symptoms because he fears losing his disability payments and returning to his stressful workplace. In most patients, multiple etiological factors appear to play a part, and the relative contribution of each may change with the passage of time. (p. 249)

There is a tendency to blame the somatizer for overreporting of the symptoms. That emotional problems are viewed as a moral failing (for example, "strong people can solve their own problems") also brings shame to anyone who acknowledges having such.

Certain economic realities tend to complicate matters. Insurance carriers are typically willing to pay for treatment if a condition is deemed to be "medical," but not if the same condition is diagnosed as "psychological." Even with the best policies these days, coverage for mental illnesses, especially those not requiring hospitalization or other psychiatric intervention, is considerably less than for comparable medical illnesses.

This means that people who actually are psychology patients end up being seen within the medical system—a potentially troubling experience for everyone concerned. Accordingly, somatizing patients don't improve, doctors feel thwarted, and insurance carriers are disinclined to continue paying for treatment that shows no results.

From a strictly financial viewpoint, somatizing disorders have traditionally generated income for physicians. Patients' persistent medical complaints keep them returning for medical services because their complaints aren't being addressed. With today's managed care and cost limitations, these same disorders have turned into economic liabilities for the medical system, which is carefully scrutinized into containing costs. This has only intensified the medical system's negative reactions toward somatizing patients.

The net result of these social forces is that patients and doctors end up "medicalizing" psychological problems. This gives us the phenomenon of somatization and, in some cases, health anxiety syndrome.

Somatoform Disorders

Somatization is often discussed within the context of *somatoform disorders*, which are diagnosable psychiatric disorders characterized by physical symptoms that suggest the presence of, but aren't completely explained by, a verifiable, underlying physical condition. In other words, the physical symptoms or their severity and duration can't be completely explained by an underlying physical condition. As the name implies, somatoform disorders (from the Greek *soma*, meaning "body") exist at the "body-mind interface" where the body and mind influence one another. Conflicts within the mind influence the brain into directing the body to react. And the brain, in ways only recently outlined and still not fully understood, sends signals into the person's conscious awareness indicating a serious problem in the body.

If you have health anxiety, you might experience one or more of the following characteristics resembling a somatoform disorder, including:

- Physical complaints indicating medical ailments that, following exhaustive medical investigations, seem to have no serious, verifiable, or pertinent disease process that explains them

- Psychological conflicts that appear to be central to the presence of the ailments

- Malfunction in your ability to live, love, or work

What about hypochondria and health anxiety syndrome? The somatoform disorder that most closely resembles health anxiety is *hypochondria* (or "hypochondriasis"), which accounts for about 4 to 9 percent of patients seeking services from general medical practices (American Psychiatric Association 1994). This diagnosable disorder involves a persistent (more than six months' duration), unrealistic preoccupation with the possibility of having a serious disease. Hence, common and normal sensations are misinterpreted as abnormal and as signs of serious disease. As one patient noted:

When I get even the smallest ache or pain, my brain
immediately decides it's a sign of impending disaster.
For example, the other night my toe was hurting, and
in true fashion I worried all night that I'd have to have
it amputated. I know it's ridiculous, so I keep fighting my
tendency to magnify things out of proportion.

There is no known, direct cause of hypochondria, but it frequently develops in people who've experienced or witnessed a major
disease firsthand. Some medical evidence also suggests that hypo-
chondriacs might, in fact, be physically ill—though not from the diseases they fear. Instead, their problems can be brought on by
chemical imbalances in the brain from such factors as stress, early
learning, or heredity. Whatever the cause, three mechanisms consistently play a role in the development of true hypochondria:

- Preoccupation with and amplification of bodily symptoms

- A need to be sick and taken care of

- Relegation to the role of "identified patient" (the one who's
  "always sick") in the hypochondriac's family system

Specific symptoms of diagnosable hypochondria usually include:

- Intense and persistent fear of serious illness that virtually
  controls all aspects of life

- Misinterpretation and exaggeration of symptoms

- Bodily symptoms that shift, change, or move to different
  parts of the body

- No discernible physical disorder that can account for the
  symptoms

- Minimal insight into the psychological nature of the
  symptoms

- Persistent refusal to accept the reassurance of several different doctors that there is no physical illness

- Impairment in life functioning due to frequent appointments
  with health-care providers or the overuse of sick days at
  work

- The disturbance lasting for a minimum of six months

Do any of these symptoms sound familiar? They should. For many sufferers of health anxiety syndrome, one or more of these symptoms are present, even though they might be of lesser intensity or of a different quality than those of full-blown hypochondriasis. For other sufferers, symptoms resembling an anxiety disorder are the more dominant.

Practical Pointer

Even though you don't have diagnosable hypochondria, as a sufferer of health anxieties you might experience one or more of the symptoms of hypochondria.

Anxiousness

All humans experience fear and anxiety. Fear involves emotional, biological, and behavioral reactions to a recognized threat (such as a prowler or a runaway vehicle). It's there to keep us safe in times of danger, and it's usually uncomfortable (except when we purposely frighten ourselves, such as when watching a scary movie or riding a roller coaster). If, for example, you're afraid of being hurt in an automobile accident, you're more likely to avoid dangerous driving situations and less likely to be reckless on the road. In other words, *adaptive anxiety* helps us be appropriately cautious in potentially dangerous situations. For example, it's adaptive to fear large animals, criminals, and other potentially dangerous situations.

Let's face it, we live in troubled times, so it's no wonder most of us have anxiety. Threats of deadly plagues, economic troubles, unemployment, and even war and terrorism have become everyday worries in this country. As an extreme example, the terrorist attacks of September 11 have left an indelible mark on us all. In the aftermath of this horrific tragedy, many people remain afraid to travel. Law-abiding Arab-Americans fear reprisal and discrimination. And many of us worry about potential chemical or biological attacks.

However, you should remember that such fear reactions are to be expected. The real psychological problem begins when *fear takes on a life of its own*—when it causes significant personal distress and interference in daily living. Such *maladaptive anxiety* causes both anguish and dysfunction; it's unrealistic and out of proportion to the actual threat of danger. For example, it's maladaptive to have panic attacks while quietly sitting at home watching television. In these instances, you have to consider the possibility of having a full-fledged *anxiety disorder*.

Anxiety Disorders

If you have health worries, you probably have one or more of the symptoms of an anxiety disorder, one of the more common psychological problems. The World Health Organization has even identified anxiety as a major affliction facing today's world.

The causes of anxiety disorders are poorly understood, but seem to include both biological and psychological factors. Biologically speaking, our thoughts and feelings can be viewed as the result of electrochemical processes in the brain. This fact, though, does little to explain the complicated interactions among neurotransmitters and neuromodulators in the brain, or about abnormal versus normal stimulation and anxiety. Psychologically speaking, anxiety is probably the result of environmental stressors (such as divorce, death, change in career) acting upon the biology of the brain. Anxiety disorders, then, can occur when the brain malfunctions or is overwhelmed by events.

What about OCD and health anxiety syndrome? Health anxiety syndrome most closely resembles the anxiety disorder obsessive-compulsive disorder. OCD is characterized by *obsessions* (recurrent and persistent thoughts, impulses, or images that are experienced as being intrusive and inappropriate) and *compulsions* (repetitive behaviors that are performed in response to an obsession). The most common obsessions have these themes:

- Fear of contamination by dirt, germs, or poisons

- Fear of having a serious illness

- Fear that one's actions will hurt other people or bring about bad things

- Inability to discard useless items (hoarding)

- Improper sexual and aggressive thoughts and images

- A need for order, symmetry, or precision

If your excessive health worries are more akin to OCD, you might find yourself thinking about germs, bodily symptoms, or diseases. You might worry about shaking hands or drinking from public water fountains. You might also want to take more showers or wash your hands frequently. Or you might avoid things, places, and situations that trigger your health anxieties in the first place, like doorknobs, public restrooms, and parties.

What about simple phobia and health anxiety syndrome? Another type of anxiety disorder that health anxiety syndrome can mimic is *simple phobia*. This disorder manifests itself as an irrational, overblown reaction to ordinarily harmless objects or situations. The most common simple phobias are those of animals, insects, blood, injury, dental procedures, driving, flying, sex, heights, and closed spaces.

It's also possible to have a simple phobia of contaminants, germs, blood, hospitals, medical instruments, injury, accidents, and illness. Undoubtedly, certain cases of health anxiety appear related to this particular form of anxiety disorder.

Practical Pointer

For many sufferers of health anxiety syndrome, one or more of the symptoms of a diagnosable anxiety disorder—especially OCD and simple phobia—are present, although the patient falls short of a full-blown diagnosis.

Causes of Health Anxiety Syndrome

Like the somatoform and anxiety disorders in general, there is no easily identified cause of health anxiety syndrome. To date, a variety of suggestions have been proposed. Some of the more popular of these include:

- Complications from physical or mental disorders

- A childhood history of actual organic illness

- A childhood history of using illness to garner attention

- Close involvement with a sick relative

- Life experiences that have caused feelings of threat and insecurity

• Depression or disruption in the usual social network (especially seen in the elderly)

From this list, it should be obvious that health worries can both be *triggered by* and *coexist with* actual physical conditions and diseases. Unfortunately, this complicates matters significantly and makes diagnosis tricky. To the medical profession's credit, teasing apart the physical and emotional components of a person's complaints can prove formidable.

Let's consider the case of David, whose multiple bouts with cancer definitely played a role in his health fears.

David is a sixty-year-old man with a lifelong history of physical symptoms, health problems, illnesses, injuries, and serious and not-so-serious diseases. According to his parents, David was often "sickly" as a child. He frequently caught colds, suffered from allergies, and had many somatic complaints. Looking back, he also frequently "used" his illnesses to get the attention of his mother (who was preoccupied herself with taking care of a terminally ill relative). In fact, the only time David's mother paid him much attention was when he wasn't well.

His older brother reports that, as a child, David also "used" somatic symptoms to avoid chores at home or help at his father's business. For example, when the father's employees would call into work sick, the boys would be called to come help. David would then suddenly develop a headache, dizziness, or other symptom. This meant his brother would have to help their father while David stayed at home in bed and enjoyed his mother's care.

At about age ten, David complained of chest problems that prompted his mother to take him to a hospital for a chest X-ray. Through either neglect or accident (and, to this day, no one knows for sure), David's chest was exposed to X-rays for over an hour. This unfortunate incident was suspected as the cause of David's breast cancer, which first appeared when David was in his late thirties. Following a radical mastectomy, David appeared to have recovered from the cancer, until several years later when the cancer reappeared as small spots on David's lungs.

Chemotherapy was given this time, and consisted not of radiation but of injections of an experimental drug designed to treat prostate cancer. Treatment lasted for several months and successfully destroyed the cancer cells.

Since that time, David has had yearly checkups, and the cancer has never reoccurred.

But David's bouts with cancer led to another, unexpected consequence: anxiety about his health, including fears of the cancer recurring. Following this second bout, he began to obsess over his physical condition. He also began to schedule frequent appointments with doctors to figure out what was wrong.

David also developed a mysterious "wooziness" that would reoccur whenever he didn't want to do something. He started spending much of his free time in bed "resting," especially when there was work to be finished, children to be driven somewhere, or shopping to be done. Not surprisingly, David's mysterious illnesses started to take a toll on the members of his immediate and extended family.

David also grumbled more and more about pain in his extremities and numerous other physical symptoms. As it tuns out, although the experimental treatment used during David's early forties cured his cancer, it also caused his spine to begin to degenerate—a sort of osteoporosis—during his fifties.

During a particularly stressful period in his working life, David complained even more about back and neck pain. He started taking several narcotic pain pills every day, and eventually scheduled two lower back surgeries. These surgeries only temporarily stopped the pain, which began moving around his body (to his legs, then his feet, to his knees, then to his neck). David's physicians agreed that David's reported pain was inconsistent with their medical conclusions.

Meanwhile, David's wife was becoming increasingly exhausted and depressed at having to deal with her husband's conditions and illnesses. And the more she tried to ignore David, the more he seemed to complain, feel "woozy," become angry, and so forth.

When he retired in his late fifties, David began scheduling even more doctor's appointments, sometimes having several in the same day. He expected his wife to handle all the medical paperwork, which was becoming increasingly complicated given the growing number of medical professionals David was seeing. He was also experiencing memory problems from years of daily narcotic intake, again placing burdens on his wife.

Whenever it was recommended that David see a mental health therapist, he would become upset and claim his problems were "everyone else's fault." He eventually tried counseling, but quit after a few sessions, arguing that he didn't need counseling because "nothing will ever change at home."

As it stands today, David continues to search for "the answer" to his health problems. He persistently worries about having another major disease, yet is frustrated with the repeated lack of medical findings. And not long ago, his wife reported that after David learned that their youngest son needs knee surgery, David began complaining of severe knee problems.

Again, health anxieties don't necessarily arise in the absence of all organic conditions. In many cases, disease phobics have a history of real diseases. This is one of the reasons why so many cases of health anxiety appear, at least initially, *not* to be clear-cut cases of either physical or emotional disturbance. And because today's medical profession tends to approach most problems from a strictly biological perspective, the usual pattern is to order a multitude of medical tests and exams in an effort to find the actual problem. Only after numerous failures to identify a physical cause does the possibility of a psychological problem enter the conversation, although most disease phobics don't care for this answer.

Stress and Inner Conflicts

As I mentioned in the Introduction, stress and unresolved conflicts do play roles in creating health anxieties. How? Stress alters your general perceptions and interpretations of life, which then trigger a variety of physical ailments, such as low back pain or respiratory problems. So, you seek help from doctor after doctor, but never feel like you've received any tangible answers—only more dead ends. This causes more stress, which causes more symptoms, which causes more stress. And so it goes until you decide to get off the roller coaster.

Unresolved psychological conflicts can also aggravate your problems. Scientists aren't sure why, but for many people who haven't dealt with their innermost conflicts, their underlying emotions, desires, and frustrations can find expression as bodily symptoms, as well as anxiety over those symptoms.

You need to remember that, while we'd all like a simple medical clarification for our health worries, biology doesn't explain everything. But neither can we ignore biology when talking about health— be it physical, mental, or both. This means your health anxieties are probably best seen as developing in response to a combination of interacting genetic tendencies and life experiences, such as a history of childhood illnesses or a major life trauma. And once activated, your health anxieties are reinforced as you repeatedly receive attention or sympathy from family, friends, neighbors, and the health-care system. (That's the *secondary gain* I mentioned earlier.) The problem, then, becomes a tenacious one—to the point that others see your so-called hypochondria as being ingrained into your personality.

In my opinion, and I'll have a lot more to say about this point in future chapters, most health anxieties are due to, and worsened by, *irrational thinking patterns.* In other words, while a number of causes like stress and pent-up emotions play a leading role in triggering uncomfortable symptoms and health worries, *health anxiety syndrome mostly has to do with the way you think about your bodily sensations, symptoms, and general health.* The good news, of course, is that you can do something about your health worries because *you can change your thinking and attitudes!*

Practical Pointer

Stress and unresolved psychological conflicts can manifest as physical symptoms—a first step in developing health anxiety syndrome. However, most health anxieties are due to, or at least worsened by, irrational thinking patterns. If you worry too much about your health, you must be willing to accept the fact that there is nothing wrong with you physically. Once you realize that your mind is doing this to your body, you'll have taken the first step on the road to recovery.

A Self-Test for Health Anxiety Syndrome

Now that we've looked at the concept of health anxiety syndrome, here is a self-test to assess to what degree, if any, you worry too much about your health. For each of the following, answer "yes" if true or "no" if false. Try to answer every question. When you're done, tally up your "yes" responses and interpret your score according to the directions at the end of the test.

1. Do you have a marked and persistent fear of germs or contracting a disease? _____ Yes _____ No

2. Do you immediately conclude that everyday physical symptoms are reflections of a serious illness? _____ Yes _____ No

3. Do you make repeated visits to doctors or other health-care providers or request multiple medical tests? _____ Yes _____ No

4. Do you "doctor shop"? _____ Yes _____ No

5. Do you leave medical appointments feeling like you've accomplished little or nothing? _____ Yes _____ No

6. Does thinking about your health usually cause you to become anxious or panicky? _____ Yes _____ No

7. Do your health worries seem unreasonable to you and/or those close to you? _____ Yes _____ No

8. Do you lose sleep over your health worries? _____ Yes _____ No

9. Do your health worries ever interfere with your daily routine, job, school, family, or social relationships? _____ Yes _____ No

10. Have doctors consistently ruled out a physical cause for your symptoms, even though you continue to complain and request additional physical examinations, tests, second opinions, etc.? _____ Yes _____ No

11. If a medical condition or disease is brought to your attention (through the media or someone you know), do you worry about getting it yourself? _____ Yes _____ No

12. If you feel sick and another person tells you that you look fine, do you become irritated? _____ Yes _____ No

13. Are you troubled by too many pains or aches? _____ Yes _____ No

14. Do you feel other people don't take your health problems seriously enough? _____ Yes _____ No

15. Do you ever distrust your doctor when he/she tells you there's nothing physically wrong with you? ____ Yes ____ No

16. Do you ever avoid touching objects or shaking people's hands for fear of germs or contracting a disease? ____ Yes ____ No

17. Do you ever have trouble ignoring your physical symptoms? ____ Yes ____ No

18. Do you ever engage in rituals, like washing your hands many times every day, as a way of dealing with your fears of contamination? ____ Yes ____ No

19. Do you overexercise because you worry you won't stay in shape? ____ Yes ____ No

20. Do you get apprehensive when you miss one or two days of exercise? ____ Yes ____ No

22. Do you obsess over diet, fat, vitamin supplements, or nutrition? ____ Yes ____ No

23. Do you use special air filters at home to eliminate germs from the air? ____ Yes ____ No

24. Are you afraid of dying from a serious disease? ____ Yes ____ No

25. Do people ever tell you that you "use" your symptoms and illnesses to get attention, sympathy, or something else? ____ Yes ____ No

The more "yes" responses you have, the more likely it is that you have health anxiety syndrome:

- A score of 0–5 indicates little or no health anxiety

- A score of 5–20 indicates possible health anxiety

- A score over 20 indicates probable health anxiety

Whatever your score is, you'll want to continue reading *Stop Worrying About Your Health!* You can also talk with a licensed clinician if you want more information.

For Personal Reflection

Throughout this book, I've included numerous self-assessment exercises entitled, "For Personal Reflection" and "Questions for Thought." These are designed to help you reflect on your own experience as it relates to what you've just read. Many people find it helpful to write their responses to these exercises and questions in a journal— a practice that I recommend.

Based on your results from the self-test for health anxiety syndrome, do you worry too much about your health? If so, when did you first realize your tendency to do this? What were the circumstances? Or are you reading this because someone you love or know is preoccupied with his or her health?

Conclusions

Health anxiety syndrome involves fixation on bodily symptoms and fear of illness. It's an irrational fear of physical disease regardless of medical assurances of health. In some cases, health anxiety syndrome more closely resembles hypochondria, while in other cases it more closely resembles obsessive-compulsive disorder or a simple phobia. Whatever their manifestation, health anxieties can cause anguish and even impairment in many important areas of life.

It's my professional opinion that you *can* worry too much about your health without necessarily having a mental disorder. In the feature at the end of chapter 5, I discuss some of the intricacies of how psychologists and psychiatrists make diagnoses. But first, I'd like us to think about health anxiety syndrome within an important context—that of mind-body psychology.

Feature: Health Anxiety
and Medical Students

If you think you worry too much about your health, you're not alone. One group that appears to experience a higher-than-average rate of occurrence of health anxiety is medical students.

It's well known that doctors-to-be frequently develop symptoms of illness and even serious disease phobias—a phenomenon known as "medical student's disease," "medical-student-itis," and "medical student hypochondria." These students often end up seeking reassurances from their own physician, having multiple medical examinations, and scheduling unnecessary lab tests. The distress of health anxiety syndrome in medical students can also interfere with their studies and training.

Why does medical student hypochondria happen? One explanation has to do with the heightened awareness of disease and germs that medical students have because of their constant exposure to sick people. Another is that intensive medical training brings out latent health fears that might already be present. Another explanation is that trainee doctors who incorrectly think they have a disease often enjoy secondary gain—whether they realize it or not—in the form of more attention and excused absences from their instructors and supervisors.

Question for Thought: Have you ever read about a disease or illness, only to find yourself thinking you have the same?

2

The Power of
Mind-Body Psychology

Thoughts are energy. And you can make your world or
break your world by thinking.

—Susan Taylor

Do any of the following comments ring true for you?

My body just won't do what my mind tells it to. No matter how hard I try to relax, I just can't.

When I get upset about something, within seconds my stomach turns nauseous. It's like there's a wire connecting my head to my gut. I'll even vomit if the stress is bad enough.

I've suffered from migraines for years. Nothing I do seems to help, although they're always worse when I'm stressed out or don't get enough sleep.

My allergies got better after I quit my job and went to work somewhere else!

The more I worry about getting sick, the more I seem to get sick!

If you've ever had thoughts like these, you're in good company. Like yourself, millions of people experience a direct relation between what they think (or sense, perceive, pay attention to) and what they feel in their body.

As I suggested in the last chapter, health anxiety syndrome is fundamentally a "mind-body" problem. By this I mean your health worries always include both physical and mental components; so it isn't "all in your head" as some non-sufferers might argue. There is always a connection between the two, even though your mind plays a primary role in starting, maintaining, and remedying health anxiety syndrome.

Therefore, our mind-body model has implications for both explaining and treating your health worries. In this chapter, we'll explore some of the basics of *mind-body psychology*—a specialty of psychology devoted to understanding the links between mental and physical events. I'll explain how this specialty includes perspectives and techniques that effectively treat many medical and behavioral problems. I'll also introduce you to the *biopsychosocial model*, which explains how mental phenomena involve biological, psychological, and social influences. According to this biopsychosocial model, problems like health anxiety syndrome are best seen as many-sided problems involving various levels of interaction among the different influences.

What Is Mind-Body Psychology?

It's easier to relax while on vacation than in the midst of the daily hassles of life. We all know that stresses, failings, and disappointments can drain your physical energy to the point that a simple allergen like pollen can reduce your mental and emotional stamina. It's easy to see that the mind and the body are interrelated.

A Little History

Of course, questions related to the body and the mind are nothing new, and are not of exclusive interest to those of us living in the twenty-first century. The issue has piqued the curiosity of great thinkers for centuries.

For instance, in the disciplines of philosophy and psychology (which prior to 1879 were generally considered to be one and the same), *mind-body dualism* refers to any theory that the mind and body are distinct forms of matter, separate natures, or unrelated substances. Hence, a "dualist" would disapprove of any assumption that equates the mind with the brain, which is a physical mechanism.

This modern question of the relationship of mind and body stems from the writings of seventeenth-century French mathematician and philosopher Rene Descartes. With his famous phrase, "Cogito, ergo sum" (Latin for "I think, therefore I am"), Descartes conceptualized the mind as an immaterial substance that engages in the activities of reasoning, thinking, imagining, willing, and feeling. He also saw the mind as entirely separate from the body. Among the difficulties of dualism as a concept is its innate inability to define precisely what a mental substance—a thinking, metaphysical "essence"—actually is. These kinds of criticisms have led modern theorists to abandon the theory of dualism in favor of more scientific models.

Interestingly, no metaphysical problem is discussed more vigorously today than that of the complex interactions of mind and body. In fact, modern-day scientists have added their own spin to this issue as they've become increasingly fascinated with the idea that our thoughts, attitudes, emotions, behaviors, and health are all affected by the others. Such intrigue with the so-called mind-body connection led to the development of a new branch of psychology known as mind-body psychology (also called *health psychology, behavioral medicine,* or *psychosomatic medicine*), as well as a new branch of medicine known as psychoneuroimmunology. Of these two broad categories, mind-body psychology as a scientific discipline is the more inclusive in its study of mind-body-spirit events, while psycho-neuroimmunology is more specific in its study of the links between the immune system and emotions.

The Bottom Line?

The interdependence of the mind and body is evident in everything we do, from cutting the grass, to loving our pets, to mastering a musical instrument. In fact, it's difficult *not* to find these links in our lives, mainly because we humans are biological, mental, social, emotional, and spiritual beings. It's just that the same mind-body interactions that bring us joy in life also pose a special problem for sufferers of health anxiety syndrome.

This emphasis on the mutual reliance among your attitudes, emotions, and behaviors means that *you can choose to make a difference in your recovery from health anxieties*. It means that by changing the way you look at your world, you can influence the status of your health and the course of your life. I'll speak more to this process of restructuring your thoughts—a process known as *cognitive reframing*—in chapters 3 and 4.

Practical Pointer

Mind-body psychology is a scientific discipline that seeks to understand and explain how the mind and body interrelate.

What Do Mind-Body Psychologists Do?

An important aspect of mind-body psychology is its focus on the effect that psychological factors have on health. Mind-body psychologists typically study why people become sick, how their behavior influences their health, and how they stay free of sickness. These psychologists also study many other health-related topics, such as the promotion of fitness, instruction in stress management, and the enhancement of health-care policies and services, to name only a few.

We'll now look at some of the effects that psychological factors can have on physical disorders, how Type A behaviors and personality traits can influence health, and a few methods to improve both physical and mental health. Then we'll examine how mind-body principles apply to health anxiety syndrome.

The Mind, Physical Conditions, and Stress

The American Psychiatric Association's *Diagnostic and Statistical Manual of Mental Disorders* (DSM) is the standard diagnostic reference used by mental health professionals. This book lists the criteria needed for patients to qualify for any particular psychiatric diagnosis. It also defines each mental disorder, lists its associated features, and provides a variety of other descriptors.

The authors of the DSM use the phrase "psychological factors affecting medical conditions" to refer to those attitudes and emotions that contribute to the start or worsening of physical conditions. (This is in contrast to more popular terminology like "psychosomatic illness.") The DSM lists many psychological factors that influence health; some of these include psychological symptoms, personality traits, mental disorders, unhealthy behaviors, and stress (which seems to be the common link among all or most mind-body problems). The DSM also lists some of the physical conditions most commonly affected by psychological factors; some of these include gastrointestinal (for example, stomach and intestines), cardiovascular (heart), dermatological (skin), neurological (nervous system), pulmonary (lungs), urogenital (urinary and reproductive), and rheumatological (joints and bones) conditions.

Below are some additional disorders that mind-body psychologists have found to be especially intriguing.

Migraine headaches. These extremely painful, vascular (involving blood vessels) headaches are probably the most common mind-body problem, affecting up to 10 percent of the American population (Castleman 2000). A migraine is usually caused by enlarged (dilated) arteries under the scalp; these put pressure on pain-sensitive nerves in the scalp. The resulting pain is typically described as "throbbing" or "excruciating," depending on the sufferer. "Needle-like" pain behind one or both eyes, visual disturbances, nausea, vomiting, and sleepiness are also common. One theory is that migraine headache sufferers have blood vessels that are extremely sensitive to stress and subsequent nervous system activity. Given the obvious role of stress in the majority of migraine cases, treatments include stress-reduction techniques like relaxation training and biofeedback, as well as medications.

Ulcers. Ulcers involve irritation, even tiny holes, in the lining of the stomach or duodenum (a part of the small intestine). Apparently linked in many cases with the presence of the bacterium *H. pylori* in the stomach, ulcers are definitely worsened by stress, anxiety, anger, uncontrollable life events, aspirin or ibuprofen, smoking, and overconsumption of coffee. Why? When confronted with stressors, the nervous system reduces the amount of blood supplying the protective mucus layer of the stomach, which leads to increases in the secretion of stomach acid. Today, doctors typically treat ulcers with antibiotics (to eliminate the *H. pylori* bacterium), as well as with acid-neutralizing medications, changes in lifestyle habits and diet, and relaxation exercises to reduce stress.

Allergies. Allergic reactions can have many triggers. Some of the more common ones include food, pollens, medications, clothing, dust, cosmetics, and other irritants in the home and at work. Psychological factors can also cause or exacerbate allergies. Stress is a well-documented trigger of allergic reactions.

Bronchial asthma. This is a respiratory disorder typified by increased sensitivity of the lungs, which results in a narrowing of the airways. Some authorities argue that asthma, while largely brought on by biological causes, is mostly affected by psychological and social stressors. In addition to taking medications, asthmatic persons are often helped by practicing stress-management techniques and avoiding allergens.

Hypertension. Popularly known as high blood pressure, hypertension is a type of cardiovascular disorder that involves increases in blood pressure above satisfactory levels (generally above a diastolic pressure of 90 and a systolic pressure of 160). In many instances of hypertension, anxiety and stress are critical mediating factors. Specifically, stress increases sympathetic nervous system arousal, which prompts sharp increases in blood pressure. Continued sympathetic activity and arterial constrictions can lead to high blood pressure in both susceptible (including those with a family history of hypertension, African Americans, and others) and nonsusceptible persons.

Coronary heart disease. Coronary heart disease (CHD) is the number one cause of all deaths in the United States (Balch and Balch 1997). CHD refers to any condition that causes a narrowing of the coronary arteries. Numerous risk factors are thought to promote

CHD, including obesity, high levels of cholesterol, high dietary fat intake, smoking, a sedentary lifestyle, hypertension, diabetes, genetics, and stress. According to the American Heart Association, stress is strongly implicated in about half of the cases of CHD. This suggests that preventing heart disease begins in the psyche. To have healthy hearts, we must change our diets, lifestyle habits, angry emotions, and negative thoughts.

Is there a connection between type A personality traits and CHD? *Undoubtedly.* Literally volumes of research papers have been published since the 1960s examining this relationship. For instance, physicians Ray Rosenman and Meyer Friedman have investigated the long-term effects of stress-causing behavior patterns on heart disease (Carmelli, Dame, Swan, and Rosenman 1991). They have found that type As are hostile, hurried, impatient, competitive, tense, and cranky. And they're twice as likely as type Bs (more relaxed persons) to develop heart disease. This is especially the case with "anger-in" type As (those who bottle up their emotions) versus "anger-out" type As (those who freely express their emotions).

Which treatments are the best for type A patterns and CHD? Stress management skills that modify the essential personality seem to predominate: instruction in how to recognize and lessen hostile overreactions, training in communication skills, training in problem-solving, relaxation exercises, cognitive therapy, and sensible goal-setting. In short, type A people can learn self-help and effective communication skills and thus reduce their risks of heart disease and other problems.

For Personal Reflection

Take a look at yourself for a moment. Do you insist that everything be done speedily and perfectly? Do you drive yourself and others too hard? Do you hate to wait at traffic lights or in grocery store or post office lines? Do you prefer to try to do several things simultaneously? Do you relish opportunities to compete with others or yourself? Do you live on a deadline and become hostile when people or situations get in your way?

If you answered "yes" to most of these questions, you're probably a type A individual. What do you think you can do to reduce your chances of heart disease or similar problems?

Physical pain. Afflicting millions of Americans at some time in their lives, pain is one of the most frequent medical and psychological complaints. It interrupts work, wreaks havoc in marriages, and makes life miserable. Pain also costs money in terms of lost time and wages, doctor visits, and pain medications. Backaches and head-aches are the most common and debilitating forms of pain in this country. As a mind-body problem, the experience of pain is associated with stress levels, although the exact physical mechanisms—muscle tension, "pinched nerves," the dilation or constriction of arteries—are not fully understood.

Not surprisingly, chronic pain often has a psychological element. This might explain why one of the best predictors of a "bad back" is job dissatisfaction and stress—not physical injury. In such cases, back pain serves as a natural and harmless (though painful) reaction to unwanted emotions. The pain helps to distract us from our woes in life. As Robert Kellner (1991) noted in his book, *Psychosomatic Syndromes and Somatic Symptoms*:

> Some patients apparently seek support from physicians,
> while others use symptoms as bodily metaphors to express
> distress, and, in others, the illness resolves a conflict or
> satisfies another need. (p. 248)

Psychological interventions in the form of relaxation training, biofeedback, and cognitive therapy can effectively reduce pain without the side effects so typical of drugs (including the risk of addiction to pain medication). Chiropractic spinal adjustments and acupuncture seem to help many people, as do aspirin, ice, heat, massage, hypnosis, imagery, stress management, and self-suggestion. As well, a positive attitude, humor, socializing, recalling fond memories, watching movies, listening to favorite music, hobbies—anything that'll act to distract you from the pain—can make your condition more tolerable. Dwelling on your pain isn't likely to help; telling yourself how unbearable and terrible the pain is will probably make it worse.

Why have I spent so much space describing these biologically oriented mind-body problems? To drive home the point that all

For Personal Reflection

What relation do you see in your own life between stress and the mind-body problems (for example, migraines, ulcers, allergies) mentioned above? What about the relation between stress and health anxiety syndrome?

mind-body problems are amenable to self-help psychological techniques that reduce stress and alter ineffective thinking patterns.

Improving Health: An Apple a Day

Earlier in this chapter, I listed several topics that mind-body psychologists emphasize: the promotion of health, the role of psychological factors in illness, the improvement of health care, and so forth. Beyond these, one of the more popular trends in health psychology these days is to teach effective personal attitudes and behaviors that will contribute to wellness.

Three means of enhancing health, whether or not you have health worries, are nutrition, exercise, and spirituality.

Nutrition

The old saying, "You are what you eat," probably rings truer than most of us want to admit. The amounts and types of food we eat strongly affect our physical and mental health. This is why mind-body psychologists look for ways to help people strengthen their health through sound nutrition and a sensible diet. Little doubt remains that specific food items play a role in certain conditions. For example, foods high in saturated fat are often related to high cholesterol, and excessive intake of salt is often related to hypertension.

Practical Pointer

One of the best nutritional strategies to reduce stress and anxiety is to eliminate (or at least severely limit) all processed sugar, caffeine, and alcohol. I've had patients who've experienced complete relief from debilitating anxiety, such as panic attacks, by following this simple method.

Exercise

Few Americans today are unaware of the importance of aerobic exercise in maintaining good health. Aerobic activities (like walking, jogging, running, cycling, swimming, dancing, and cross-country skiing) increase oxygen consumption, especially when engaged in for a sustained period of time (a minimum of fifteen minutes three times per week). The net effect is conditioning of both the coronary and respiratory systems, which leads to a variety of health benefits, including cardiovascular fitness, weight control, regulation of glucose and cholesterol levels, and stress control. Mind-body research further indicates that exercise decreases anxiety and improves mood.

While a majority of Americans understand the advantages of aerobics, only about half of us who start an exercise program continue beyond six months. In response to such low compliance, mind-body psychologists work to improve people's attitudes about and commitment to exercise. Why? Research indicates that having a positive attitude and definable goal (such as losing fifteen pounds of fat) increases the likelihood that you'll adhere to an exercise schedule for longer than six months. Unfortunately, for most of us, awareness of the need for aerobic activity and actually committing to regular exercise are not one and the same.

Spirituality

Ask anyone who is religious, and they'll tell you that good health is definitely related to spirituality and its fruits, which reportedly include peace, love, self-acceptance, faith, hope, responsibility, joy, openness, charity, expression of feelings, and visualization of healing. I'll have more to say about the role of spirituality in overcoming health anxiety syndrome in chapter 7. But for the moment, it's helpful to remember that many people claim victory over their health worries following a spiritual experience, "awakening," or "epiphany."

Stress and the General Adaptation Syndrome

As I've implied throughout this book, excessive stress plays a unique role in human misery. You could even say that stress is a primary operating factor in most mind-body problems.

Experts often describe stress in terms of the *general adaptation syndrome*, which is explained in detail in Hans Selye's (1976) book, *The Stress of Life*. Briefly, his model takes into account the biological reactions that occur in response to sustained and unrelenting stress. Specifically, Selye has identified three stages in a typical stress reaction, with each stage leading to increased susceptibility to illness and even death. Selye's three stages are:

*Stage 1: **Alarm*** When we experience a physical or emotional stressor, the body triggers an immediate set of reactions to counteract the stressor. Because the immune system quickly becomes depressed, our usual levels of resistance are compromised, which increases our susceptibility to infection. We typically recover rapidly when the stressor isn't severe or long-term.

*Stage 2: **Resistance*** If, on the other hand, the stress continues, our immune system must work harder to keep up with the continued demands placed on it. For a while, we can become resistant to stress. But our resolve can't last forever. This is the time to combat the stress by practicing stress management or seeking a change in scenery. The problem at this stage is failing to do anything about our stress because we believe we're not susceptible to its effects.

*Stage 3: **Exhaustion*** Because the body is unable to maintain the resistance needed to battle long-term stress, we inevitably lose our resistance. Even though one person might be more or less resistant to stress than another, nearly everyone's immunity will eventually break down from prolonged demands. When this happens, organ systems and immunity begin to fail, and we fall victim to disease. Stress disrupts the natural balance—the homeostasis—that is crucial for our good health.

Most experts agree that Selye's general adaptation syndrome clarifies how stress can prove such an ample source of health troubles. Stress is one of the most significant factors in lowering resistance and triggering the various mechanisms involved in the disease process. However, by learning stress management and relaxation procedures, you can improve your chances of keeping your overall physical and psychological well-being. I'll have more to say about stress management in chapter 5.

For Personal Reflection

Have poor nutrition, lack of exercise, an absence of spirituality, and/or lack of stress management ever increased your anxieties about your own health? What can you do to reverse such negative trends in your life?

The Big Mystery

Some estimates are that as many as 80 percent of all major illnesses are related to stress (Balch and Balch 1997). This statistic alone should indicate the need for health psychologists to study the role of stress in diverse physical conditions, including migraines, CHD, hypertension, immune disorders, and even cancer. Information gleaned from this type of research could prove useful in determining which mind-body approaches are the most useful for mind-body and stress-related difficulties.

What are we to think about individuals for whom a disease can't be easily identified? Why is discomfort experienced when there are no apparent bodily impairments? One possible answer is that our modern technology (including MRIs, CAT scans, EEG, EKG, and X-rays) isn't sensitive enough to locate minute biochemical abnormalities that cause certain types of discomfort or impairment. After all, medical instruments only measure what they're designed to measure. In the case of health anxiety syndrome, it could be that the symptoms are due to a microscopic biochemical malfunctioning related to subtle chemical or electrical balancing—one that can't yet be detected by our science.

Another, more plausible answer is that the discomfort isn't detectable by physical tests because it isn't a physical problem. Rather, the discomfort is generated in the mind. In other words, the problem is mental and not physical; the mind is responsible for the experienced physical ailments.

Of course, no single, corresponding brain structure is responsible for any particular mind-body problem. Modifying hormone levels or stimulating certain brain structures can bring about changes in levels of emotional tolerance, but it's only a generalized response. In other words, scientists haven't yet discovered an exact one-on-one relationship between areas of the brain and mental events. It may be that none exists; only time and a great deal of research will tell us for sure. So, for now, it's incorrect to conclude that exact biochemical mechanisms can account for exact thoughts, emotions, or behaviors.

Moreover, because the entire question of mind-body psychology involves subjective theories and methods, no physical object or mechanism is available to manipulate using the scientific method. This is one important reason why it's nearly impossible to identify a precise correlation between each brain function and particular human behaviors and mental processes. Instead, we have to rely on personal feedback and other self-report measures to gain additional insights into mind-body phenomena.

Thus far, we've looked at some of the basic principles of mind-body psychology. To more fully appreciate the complexities of health anxiety syndrome, though, it's a good idea to think about this syndrome from another perspective. Given my preference for holistic (multidimensional) models to explain life, I've chosen the biopsychosocial perspective for this purpose.

What Is the Biopsychosocial Perspective?

My description of health anxiety syndrome—an excessive sensitivity to symptoms and fear of disease—is based on my observations of the mutual interdependence of biological, psychological, and social influences. These three interacting influences form the essence of the *biopsychosocial perspective*, which attributes mind-body phenomena to multiple causes. (In contrast to the biopsychosocial perspective is the *reductionist perspective*, which reduces mind-body phenomena to a single, often simplistic, cause.)

Let's consider an example of applying the biopsychosocial model to health worries. Some people find it difficult or impossible to touch anything or be around other people for fear of catching germs. This form of health anxiety could be the result of any of a number of causes, including:

- Injunctions, or messages received during childhood (for example, that germs are always deadly)

- Poor understanding of disease processes

- Fear of death

- Fear of going crazy or doing something stupid in front of others

- Fear of social interactions

- Chemical imbalances in the brain

- Intense stress at work or home that is transformed into physical symptoms

- Irrational thinking patterns

As a real-life example of how interacting biological, psychological, and social processes can cause chronic health worries, Bob was raised to believe "strong boys" never get sick. They stay well, do their chores, and don't complain about aches or pains. But because he experiences distress at the thought of catching germs and becoming sick (psychological), Bob obsesses over his health, which distracts him from fully immersing himself in his work and family life (social).

In time, his nervous system becomes so aroused that relaxing and even sleeping become difficult, which causes his stress levels to continue to rise (biological). Because Bob can't concentrate on his job or anything else, he becomes hyper-alert to everyday bodily sensations (biological), and then catastrophizes about contracting a deadly disease (psychological). Becoming irritated about his inability to break free from his health obsessions (psychological), Bob begins to make excessive demands of his wife by requiring her to repeatedly clean the house, which inadvertently creates a hostile home environment that further contributes to Bob's troubles (social). Bob also phones and e-mails his physician several times a day, to the point that his doctor will no longer return his calls or schedule appointments for him (social).

Get the picture? Bob doesn't present a simple predicament. He has multiple factors—psychology, biology, and environment—that all interact to produce an uncomfortable situation. Keeping in mind the entire picture of Bob's circumstances, a therapist might choose to help Bob by first attacking his most prominent issues—in this case, his distorted thinking about germs—followed by treatment for the remainder of his problems.

To flesh out our biopsychosocial model of mind-body psychology in general, and health anxiety syndrome in particular, I now present each of three major perspectives of the model, as well as various perspectives that fall under each category.

Practical Pointer

The biopsychosocial model is a means of conceptualizing life events from a holistic (multidimensional) point of view. This model recognizes the interactions of biology, psychology, and environment in influencing most every aspect of life.

Biological Perspectives in Mind-Body Psychology

The biological perspectives are primarily concerned with the effects of biological and physical processes on a person's overall functioning. Without a doubt, the field of mind-body psychology is moving in the direction of the biological perspectives, especially as the physiological sciences continue to make impressive strides in the understanding of the biochemical and neural bases of behavior. However, we mustn't forget the role that psychology plays in physical processes. For example, although exploratory surgery to discover the causes of a patient's chest pain is a medical procedure, it is inseparable from numerous complex attitudinal, social, legal, moral, and ethical considerations. As John Sarno (1991), author of *Healing Back Pain: The Mind-Body Connection*, wrote:

> All physicians should be practitioners of "holistic medicine" in the sense that they recognize the interaction between mind and body. To leave the emotional dimension out of the study of health and illness is poor medicine and poor science. (p. xi)

The biological perspectives include the biochemical and psychiatric perspectives.

The Biochemical Perspective

At the heart of the *biochemical perspective* is the belief that all aspects of human functioning are reflections of biochemical processes. According to this model, mind-body problems are 99 percent the result of chemical imbalances or physical diseases. Biological therapists, including some physicians, treat mind-body problems by attempting to correct or reverse impaired biological processes, with little or no regard for psychological or social influences. For example, biological therapies for stress-related headaches might include drug therapy with muscle relaxants or anti-anxiety agents, but no counseling or relaxation exercises.

Two popular subcategories of the biochemical perspective are the *neural* and *genetic perspectives*. According to the *neural perspective*, all human behaviors, thoughts, and emotions have a basis in nervous system activity. The person with health anxiety, then, is seen as experiencing malfunctioning neural processes. While the actions of nerves are fairly well understood, the functioning of the nervous system as a whole in controlling behavior is not.

A slight variation on the neural perspective is the emerging field of *social neuroscience*, which combines biological and environmental approaches to explaining various phenomena. Social neuroscientists study such wide-ranging topics as love, stress, dietary habits, interpersonal violence, discrimination, and the biopsychosocial roots of illness.

Proponents of the *genetic perspective* contend that all or most aspects of human functioning are genetically determined prior to birth. Nearly all cells of the body have twenty-three pairs of *chromosomes*, the structures that contain genetic material. Within each pair, one chromosome is received from the father and the other from the mother. Chromosomes contain genes, the "blueprint" information about the structure and functioning of the body. Your experience of health anxiety syndrome, for example, could be seen as an expression of your genetic predisposition to exaggerate the seriousness of bodily symptoms.

The Psychiatric Perspective

The *psychiatric perspective* has as its basis the biochemical perspective and one or more of the psychological perspectives, described below. For a psychiatrist (who has earned the M.D. degree) using the Freudian (psychoanalytic) model, for instance, mind-body problems might be viewed as the result of both biochemical imbalances and repressed desires or conflicts. Treatment, then, might include both drug therapy to correct chemical imbalances and psychoanalysis to help lift the patient's repression. Although today's psychiatrists generally consider biological, unconscious, and psychosocial causes to be of equal importance, traditional psychiatry has relied heavily on classical Freudian theory. People often confuse the psychiatric perspective with one or more of the psychological perspectives. These differ primarily in the psychiatric perspective's heavy focus on both biochemical and mental processes.

Psychological Perspectives in Mind-Body Psychology

Those who favor *psychological perspectives* examine how thoughts, attitudes, emotions, and behaviors accumulated from a lifetime of experiences affect human functioning. As such, psychologists (who have earned the Ph.D. or other doctoral degree) are concerned with:

- Opinions ("I believe I'm a bad person because I always seem to be sick!")

- Willingness to discuss and process emotions ("My husband might reject me if I tell him how I really feel")

- Patterns of normal and abnormal behavior

- How health-related problems develop

- Techniques to influence these areas

Four psychological perspectives that relate to health worries include the *psychodynamic, cognitive behavioral, existential-humanistic,* and *systems perspectives.*

The Psychodynamic Perspective

Based on Freudian theory, the *psychodynamic perspective* is the view that an individual's unconscious motivations and desires determine how he or she interacts in the world. This perspective is similar to the traditional psychiatric perspective, but differs in its focus on psychological rather than biological influences. For example, traditional psychiatric treatment of *body dysmorphic disorder* (the perception and fear that one or more parts of your body are "out of proportion," such as believing you have gigantic arms) might include drug therapy, whereas psychodynamic therapy wouldn't. Both approaches, however, often reflect common methods of Freudian interpretation. A Freudian psychiatrist and a psychodynamic psychologist might consider a man with body dysmorphic disorder to have deep-seated conflicts about "unacceptable" sexual desires, which lead to a "symptom" that prevents him from acting out his fantasies.

Practical Pointer

Many people confuse psychiatrists with psychologists. Psychiatrists earn a medical degree and prescribe medications, while psychologists earn a graduate degree and don't prescribe medications. Both are licensed professionals who use a variety of counseling methods.

The Cognitive Behavioral Perspective

A purely *behavioral perspective* of mental functioning holds that most, if not all, mental processes are directly related to physical phenomena. As such, *behaviorists* (professionals who use behavioral techniques to treat problems) are primarily concerned with the roles that behavior and learning play in a person's life. They base their position on *learning theory*, a psychological theory holding that changes in behavior occur as a result of experience. Many psychological disorders and other problems (for example, smoking, overeating) can be treated successfully with behavior therapy.

For Personal Reflection

Injunctions are early childhood messages that we receive from our parents, teachers, and other authority figures. Think back for a minute and recall your childhood. List five injunctions that you recall receiving about health and disease.

1.

2.

3.

4.

5.

"Strict" behaviorists like B. F. Skinner have argued that cognitive (thinking) activity is relatively unimportant when studying behavior. In recent decades, researchers like David Barlow have challenged this view, leading to what some behavioral scientists have labeled the "cognitive revolution"—widespread acknowledgment of the role that cognitive processes play in affecting behavior and emotions.

Central to the *cognitive perspective* is the idea that thought processes significantly affect daily living. In other words, your *perception* of events is of critical importance, not necessarily the events themselves. And by manipulating these perceptions, it becomes possible to diminish discomfort and pain.

Many experts believe the learning perspective is incomplete if the role of cognition is ignored. This position has given rise to the *cognitive behavioral perspective*, which incorporates both learning and cognitive theories. One example of a comprehensive model of cognitive behaviorism is Albert Ellis' *rational-emotive-behavior therapy* (REBT), a type of therapy for eliminating irrational beliefs.

Besides proving useful for dealing with issues of everyday living, REBT has been successfully applied to numerous clinical problems. I'll have much more to say in the next two chapters about the power of cognitive behavioral therapies for overcoming health anxiety syndrome.

The Existential-Humanistic Perspective

The *existential-humanistic perspective* stresses the importance of immediate experience, self-acceptance, and self-actualization. Being aware of feelings is an important aspect of this perspective. Psychologically speaking, focusing too much on the past or future detracts from the present, and this can be a cause of mental problems. In contrast, being self-accepting can do much to promote calm and self-fulfillment in life. If you experience health anxiety syndrome, learning to accept yourself as you are—including any health complaints—can do much to alleviate your worries of contracting a deadly disease.

The Systems Perspective

The great majority of us exist as members of one or more social groups. The *systems perspective* is concerned with how these different social groups interrelate and affect individuals, couples, and families. The most common social systems are family, school, work, community, and religious systems.

Many of us receive irrational or conflicting messages about health from our parents, schools, and the media. Knowing which system gave what message is both enlightening and helpful for challenging these messages. Furthermore, identifying and analyzing how social systems interact is basic to understanding human behavior. Consider a child who persistently visits the school nurse complaining of a variety of vague symptoms. She could be doing so in response to problems at home, such as trouble getting along with her step siblings.

Another important aspect of the systems perspective that relates to health anxiety involves secondary gain, or the benefits (such as attention, sympathy, getting out of obligations) that become associated with the "sick role" within a particular social system. If you suffer from health anxiety syndrome, you'd best not ignore the role that secondary gain plays in your continuing to be ill. (Try asking your loved ones if they think you ever receive any benefits from being sick, and see what they say!)

For Personal Reflection

Why do you think secondary gain plays such an important role in health anxiety syndrome?

Social Perspectives in Mind-Body Psychology

What is typical for a particular group of people is only one aspect of the *social perspectives*, which are concerned with social and cultural influences and values. Two social perspectives that relate to mind-body problems are the *statistical* and *religious perspectives*.

The Statistical Perspective

The *statistical perspective* is based on the frequency of occurrence of an attitude or practice within a society. Although extremes occur within any group, statistical measurement is concerned with the characteristics of the largest number of members, in other words, the "average" members' characteristics. For example, when you have a headache, it's statistically *possible* that you have an inoperable brain tumor, but it's also highly *improbable*.

The Religious Perspective

The *religious perspective* deals with the effects that religious doctrines, scriptures, and spirituality have on individuals and society. For those of us raised in a religious environment, the teachings, morals, and values set forth by organized religion play a powerful role in life, be it healthy, harmful, or neutral. For example, some religious groups oppose mental health counseling altogether, claiming counseling and spiritual guidance from religious leaders is the preferred or even the only alternative. Others teach that it's wrong to go to a doctor when you're sick, while still others refuse blood transfusions, even in medical emergencies. Excessive mental battering from anti-medical and anti-psychology religious groups can play a part in your eventual succumbing to health anxiety.

Conclusions

Mind-body psychology is a scientific discipline devoted to exploring how closely interconnected the human mind and body are. While this chapter might seem a bit theoretical to some readers, I felt it necessary to include some background in mind-body psychology before proceeding.

We've seen how certain problems that appear to be physical are, in actuality, psychological problems. The management of such problems, then, primarily rests in the realm of the mind, not in the realm of general medicine. We've also seen how important it is to look at mind-body problems from a holistic, biopsychosocial perspective.

Health anxiety syndrome exists at the level of the mind-body interface, and is a true reflection of how the mind and body can become at odds with each other.

Now that we've laid a theoretical foundation for thinking about mind-body problems, let's apply what we've learned to understanding the irrational thinking that underlies excessive health worries.

Feature: A Mind-Body Crisis in Public Restrooms

According to Steven Soifer's (2001) book, *Shy Bladder Syndrome*, an excellent example of a mind-body problem is *paruresis*, which is informally known as *shy bladder syndrome, bashful bladder syndrome, pee-phobia,* and *bashful kidneys*. This common but little-discussed condition involves an inability to urinate in public restrooms (or any place where other people might overhear). Paruresis is primarily due to psychological causes (such as fears of criticism), but can also be influenced by physical ones (an enlarged prostate gland that blocks the flow of urine) and social ones (feeling rushed in a crowded public restroom).

The social side of shy bladder syndrome is especially apparent. In its most severe form, paruresis leaves sufferers unable to urinate under any circumstances while away from home—no matter how badly they need to urinate. In other words, the body refuses to do what the mind tells it to do. These people also do whatever they can to avoid having to use toilets away from home: they move near work, work at home, limit social outings to a few hours, and avoid fluids before traveling. Most sufferers report that the condition results in major life impairment.

Similar to other mind-body problems, treatment of paruresis involves addressing the biological, psychological, and social factors that interact to cause and maintain the condition.

Question for Thought: Why is paruresis a good example of a mind-body problem?

3

Helping Yourself with Cognitive Behavioral Therapy

Our life is what our thoughts make it.

—Marcus Aurelius

I n this chapter, we explore the theories behind the primary cause of health anxiety syndrome—cognitive distortions. I'll explain how health anxiety syndrome is related to nonsensical self-talk and behaviors, and show you how to identify your own irrational thinking.

Cognitive Behavioral Therapy

Without a doubt, the most effective approach to managing health anxiety is *cognitive behavioral therapy*, or CBT, an area of psychology concerned with why people think and act the way they do. It takes into account the primary role that illogical thinking plays in causing problems. From my point of view, CBT has a great deal to offer you in terms of the overall process of *cognitive reframing*, or improving your life by changing your thinking, attitudes, and behaviors.

The roots of the psychological self-help methods presented in this chapter go as far back as writings of the ancient Greek philosopher Epictetus. According to him and other Stoics, it's not the world that causes you problems; instead, it's how you look at the world.

This Stoic concept has endured for many centuries. For instance, William Shakespeare wrote in *Hamlet*, "There is nothing either good or bad but thinking makes it so." And John Milton wrote in *Paradise Lost*, "The mind is its own place, and in itself, can make a heaven of hell, a hell of heaven." Put simply, life's difficulties aren't caused by various external forces—like germs, incompetent doctors, and mishandled medical bills—but rather by how you react to these.

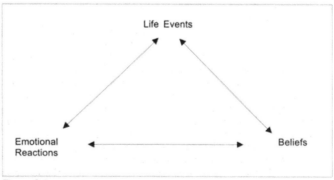

Figure 3.1

Cognitive reframing involves three major steps:

- Identifying your distorted ideas

- Challenging your distorted ideas

- Rethinking away your distorted ideas

Superficially, this might sound easy, but cognitive reframing takes some time and effort on your part. Of course, your problems didn't develop overnight; why expect them to go away easily and quickly? So, let's review *how* thinking affects life in general, and then see how CBT principles apply to health anxiety syndrome.

Basics of Cognitive Behavioral Therapy

According to the principles of CBT, beliefs, life events, emotional reactions, and behaviors all interact and affect one another, as shown in figure 3.1.

Of special importance is the direct influence that beliefs (thoughts, evaluations, attitudes) have on emotions and behaviors. From the perspective of this "Event-Belief-Reaction" model, it's your *interpretations* of people and circumstances that prompt you to feel and act the way you do—not the people or circumstances themselves. For example, Emily continually tells herself that she has a brain tumor (even when medical tests have repeatedly proven she doesn't) and terrifies herself into panic attacks, fears of dying, insomnia, and a host of other symptoms. She even berates herself and feels like a failure for not convincing her doctors or family that *she really is sick*. The more Emily engages in negative thinking, the more she believes and tells herself she isn't well, gets depressed about it, feels worse physically, and so on—all of which reinforces and perpetuates a formidable cycle of frustration, self-pity, self-defeat, increased physical discomfort, and hysteria about her health.

Most of the time when people are upset, they're telling themselves that something is *awful* or *terrible* rather than merely *inconvenient*. Psychologists refer to this process as *awfulizing* or *catastrophizing*. Put another way, the catastrophizer might decide his imperfect health is *dreadful*. Or she might conclude her life is a *disaster* when she doesn't feel the way she wants.

Whenever you believe something in life is *disastrous* or *horrible* instead of simply *unpleasant* or *unfortunate*, you've probably drawn a number of false conclusions, along the lines of these examples:

- "The situation, which is *totally bad*, makes me *utterly miserable*."

- "The condition *shouldn't exist* because *I don't like it*. I *can't tolerate* the predicament for *one minute longer*."

- "I have to find a perfect solution that will fix the situation, or else I'm a *defective person* and a *washout*."

You might also keep in mind that the vast majority of our daily problems, hassles, and disappointments come from *demanding* rather than *preferring* types of thinking. People who feel angry, anxious, nervous, irritated, or guilty do not just *desire* or *prefer* something, they usually *require*, *demand*, and *dictate* that they get what they want. As a case in point, a man might *demand* that his back pain go away, so he becomes *hostile* when it doesn't. Or he might *expect* that medical care will be *easy* and *trouble-free*, and *browbeat* himself and others when it isn't.

For people with health anxiety syndrome, these and many other irrationalities are common. This is why research has consistently shown that CBT can successfully reduce symptoms and improve functioning by:

- Teaching you to accept and redefine your experience of symptoms

- Helping you to develop active coping strategies (such as relaxation procedures for those times when you're overly stressed)

- Teaching you a new way of looking at yourself and your health

Types of Distorted Beliefs

In general, people engage in many types of nonsensical thinking. If you're preoccupied with fears of illness, you can probably relate to this. For instance, maybe you've had thoughts like:

- "I need to know with absolute certainty that I'm well."

- "If I don't take antibiotics as soon as I get sick, I'll get even sicker."

- "If my doctors were competent, they'd be able to find out what's wrong with me."

- "I must be comfortable at all times."

- "My family should pay more attention to me because I don't feel good."

Distorted beliefs are known by many names, including *cognitive distortions, irrational beliefs, crazy-makers, nonsensical notions, toxic ideas, negative automatic thoughts, negative self-talk,* and so forth. Whatever term is used, cognitive distortions of every type share some common themes. First, they usually fail the test of reason. For example, the belief, "I must enjoy perfect health," fails the test of logic, as there is no guarantee that you'll always feel well, and there is no evidence that you really *must* feel well just because you desire it. Second, unreasonable beliefs can block your ability to enjoy life because they make you so anxious. They also lead to other negative emotions, such as depression, anger, guilt, and shame, as well as destructive behaviors including social withdrawal and avoidance, aggression, drug abuse, and other self-defeating behaviors. As one client told me:

> *I'm single and lonely. I try to go out, but I just get overwhelmed with anxiety. If I manage to convince myself that I can do it—like ask a woman out on a date—then the headaches, stomachaches, allergies, and everything else under the sun start in. And then I get really down on myself. Sometimes it just doesn't seem worth it.*

Reasonable beliefs, on the other hand, help you obtain your goals and usually are sound in terms of logic and reason. They lead to such positive emotions as curiosity, excitement, joy, and happiness, as well as such constructive behaviors as approaching feared situations, tackling unpleasant but necessary chores, facing inevitable conflicts, and risking possible rejection.

Following are eleven of the most common irrational beliefs, according to Dr. Albert Ellis' (1962) classic book, *Reason and Emotion in Psychotherapy.* The idea that:

- It is a dire necessity for an adult human being to be loved or approved by virtually every significant other person in his community.

- One should be thoroughly competent, adequate, and achieving in all possible respects if one is to consider oneself worthwhile.

- Certain people are bad, wicked, or villainous and that they should be severely blamed and punished for their villainy.

- It is awful and catastrophic when things are not the way one would very much like them to be.

- Human unhappiness is externally caused and that people have little or no ability to control their sorrows and disturbances.

- If something is or may be dangerous or fearsome, one should be terribly concerned about it and should keep dwelling on the possibility of its occurring.

- It is easier to avoid than to face certain life difficulties and self-responsibilities.

- One should be dependent on others and needs someone stronger than oneself on whom to rely.

- One's past history is an all-important determiner of one's present behavior and that because something once strongly affected one's life, it should indefinitely have a similar effect.

- One should become quite upset over other people's problems and disturbances.

- There is invariably a right, precise, and perfect solution to human problems and that it is catastrophic if this perfect solution is not found. (pp. 61–88)

Some years later in his book, *How to Stubbornly Refuse to Make Yourself Miserable About Anything—Yes, Anything!,* Ellis (1988) condensed this information and proposed that all irrationality arises from three absolute *musts:*

- MUST #1: "I *must* perform well and/or win the approval of important people, or else I am an inadequate person!" (demands about self)

- MUST #2: "You *must* treat me fairly and considerately and not unduly frustrate me, or else you are a rotten individual!" (demands about others)

- MUST #3: "My life conditions *must* give me the things I want and have to have in order to keep me from harm, or else life is unbearable and I cannot be happy at all!" (demands about the world) (p. 60)

Here are thirteen additional categories of distorted beliefs collected from the writings of other psychological experts, including David Burns (1989) and Aaron Beck (1985):

- *All-or-nothing thinking:* Seeing all of life in black-or-white terms

- *Accusing:* Blaming others without the necessary evidence

- *Emotional reasoning:* Assuming one's emotional state reflects the way things really are

- *Personalizing:* Blaming oneself for some negative event

- *I-Can't-Take-It-Another-Minute-itis* (very low frustration tolerance): Easily becoming frustrated when wants aren't met

- *Damnation* (negativizing): Being excessively critical of self, others, and the world

- *Perfectionism:* Requiring that everyone and everything in the universe be flawless and without blemish

- *Mental filtering:* Focusing on specific details at the expense of other important details within a situation

- *Mind reading* (fortune telling): Presuming to know what others think, feel, or plan to do

- *Overgeneralizing:* Using words like never and always; applying the characteristics of one member to an entire group

- *Minimizing* (downplaying the positive): De-emphasizing one's positive characteristics and accomplishments

- *Magnifying* (playing up the negative; catastrophizing): Overstating the negative aspects of a situation

- *Jumping to conclusions:* Drawing conclusions about people and events without the necessary evidence

People engage in these kinds of irrationalities all of the time. Just listen to others—and to yourself—and you'll see what I mean.

For Personal Reflection

List two of your most common irrationalities for each of the following types of distortion. You can write in the book or use a separate notebook or journal.

All-or-nothing thinking:

1.

2.

Accusing:

1.

2.

Emotional reasoning:

1.

2.

Personalizing:

1.

2.

I-Can't-Take-It-Another-Minute-itis

1.

2.

Damnation:

1.

2.

Perfectionism:

1.

2.

Mental filtering:

1.

2.

Mind reading:

1.

2.

Overgeneralizing:

1.

2.

Minimizing:

1.

2.

Magnifying:

1.

2.

Jumping to conclusions:

1.

2.

Nonsensical thinking can also take the form of numerous *cognitive blocks* that interfere with healthy and intelligent living. Cognitive blocks often begin with words like, "What if . . . ?" "Oh no. . . !" "I cannot . . . !" or "How awful . . . !" Here are a few possible cognitive blocks of frustrated disease phobics:

- "I can't *ever* experience physical discomfort!"

- "Drat . . . I'm getting another headache. What if it's really serious this time, like a brain tumor?"

- "Oh no, what if I contract a serious illness? That would be *horrendous!*"

For Personal Reflection

What are your five most troublesome cognitive blocks?

1.

2.

3.

4.

5.

Now, let's take a closer look at a few of the theories and methods of the most famous all-time proponent of CBT, psychologist Albert Ellis.

Rational-Emotive-Behavior Therapy

Ellis' particular slant on CBT is known as *rational-emotive-behavior therapy* (REBT). REBT is an action-oriented approach to emotional growth that stresses your capacity for creating, altering, and controlling your emotions. REBT places a great deal of emphasis on the here and now, that is, on your current attitudes, painful emotions, and ineffective behaviors that can sabotage your happiness. Ellis believes in teaching people how to overcome the past by focusing on the present, as well as how to make effective changes in life.

Ellis labels behaviors that are "self-defeating" as "irrational," and behaviors that are "self-helping" as "rational." If you have problems, Ellis recommends you become more rational. In this way, you can increase your effectiveness and happiness at work, at home, at school, or just about anywhere else.

Like the CBT methods described in the previous section, Ellis proposes that emotional reactions aren't directly caused by events, but by one's beliefs about those events. In particular, Ellis uses an

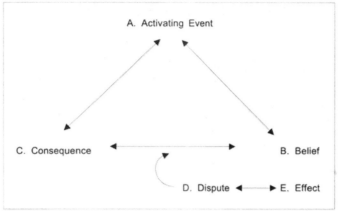

A. Activating Event

C. Consequence

B. Belief

D. Dispute

E. Effect

Figure 3.2

A-B-C model to describe the process of identifying and challenging irrational beliefs. The figure above illustrates the A-B-C theory of REBT.

In figure 3.2, A stands for "activating event," which is an external event or situation of some sort that has prompted irrationality. Here B represents "belief," C represents "upsetting emotional consequence," D represents "dispute," and E represents "new emotional consequence" or "effect."

To illustrate, let's take the example of a person with a germ phobia. Dave has an excessive fear of contracting germs from shaking other people's hands. According to REBT, A refers to the situation of touching another person, while C refers to both the anxiety expressed when thinking about or actually shaking hands, and to avoidance of the feared activity. REBT holds that it isn't A that directly causes C, but rather the B (or Bs) that Dave has about A. Moreover, A influences B in the sense that without another person's hand to shake, Dave's irrational beliefs are less likely to occur. B influences A in that whether Dave approaches A is influenced by his beliefs regarding both the appropriateness of shaking hands and his willingness to do so. C influences B in that Dave's emotions affect the likelihood of the occurrence of different types of thoughts.

The more nervous Dave is about germs, the more likely he is:

- To worry about his anxiety being seen by significant others

- To expect trouble

In a similar way, C influences A because when Dave is anxious, he might also be more likely to avoid the A of shaking hands, even if it's wise to do so (for example, when Dave's boss extends a hand in greeting). Finally, A can directly influence C, as, for example, when Dave is startled by an undesirable reaction, such as his boss' becoming insulted and angry.

We can outline our germ phobic's situation according to Ellis' A-B-C model as follows:

A. *Activating event*: Anticipating having to shake the boss' hand at an upcoming business luncheon

B. *Beliefs*:

- "I know I'll freeze up and not be able to shake his hand." (overgeneralizing)

- "If I freeze up, I won't be able to stand it. It would be awful (catastrophizing), and I'd be less of a person." (self-berating)

C. *Consequences* (emotions and behaviors):

- Extreme health anxiety

- Exacerbation of health symptoms (such as headaches, sweaty palms, ulcer pain)

- Avoiding the boss and/or the luncheon, even when it isn't politically correct to do so

D. *Disputes* (rational challenges)

- "How do I know that I'll freeze up? Maybe I will, but hopefully I won't, particularly if I work very hard at challenging my irrational beliefs."

- "If I did freeze up, I could stand it even though I wouldn't like it. It would be unfortunate but not really catastrophic."

- "How is my worth as a person determined by my ability to shake someone's hand? It isn't! At worst, it's a problem for me, but I'm not the same as my behaviors!"

In short, while REBT admits a relationship among situations, thoughts, feelings, and behaviors, at the core of Ellis' theory is the idea that *beliefs play a primary role in creating and maintaining any emotional disturbance, including health anxiety.*

Following are a few more REBT concepts that relate to self-help therapy for excessive health concerns.

Disturbance and Discomfort

Ellis proposes two essential forms of emotional disturbance that are consequences of holding onto irrational *musts* (e.g., "I must never have pain."): *ego anxiety* and *discomfort anxiety.*

Ego anxiety refers to anxiety, depression, and other emotions and behaviors that result from rating yourself as inadequate, inferior, or worthless if you don't perform certain tasks well or if you fail to obtain desired love or approval from others.

Discomfort anxiety refers to anxiety, depression, and other emotions and behaviors that result when your demands for comfort or the absence of discomfort aren't met. Health anxiety is primarily an expression of discomfort anxiety, even though ego and discomfort disturbances often occur together.

According to Albert Ellis (1982):

> Whenever ego anxiety is profound, it leads to such heightened feelings of discomfort (such as panic, horror, or terror) that people conclude that these feelings absolutely *must* not, *should* not exist, that it is awful if they do, and that life is too much a hassle for them to experience almost any enjoyment whatever under these conditions. They then are in the throes of discomfort anxiety. And whenever extreme discomfort anxiety or feelings of low frustration tolerance exist, most humans sooner or later tend to put themselves down for having and indulging in such feelings. (p. 35)

Self-Acceptance

For practical reasons, REBT promotes *self-acceptance* rather than *self-esteem.* According to Ellis, self-esteem involves self-rating (for example, "I'm a good person when I feel well, display positive characteristics, or get what I want. I'm less of a person when I feel lousy, display negative characteristics, or fail to get what I want"). Self-acceptance involves receiving yourself as you are today.

REBT urges self-acceptance rather than self-rating for several reasons. First, human beings are "in-process" and constantly changing. Second, there's no accurate way to measure human characteristics. Third, it's impossible to keep track of all personality characteristics and behaviors.

Anti-Catastrophizing

Ultimately, you learn from REBT that nothing in life is catastrophic. Many stressors, like chronic pain or a disability, are plainly unfortunate and bad, but none of them is truly awful, horrible, or terrible. You need to accept this tenet of REBT if any of the other described techniques or philosophical ideas are to prove beneficial.

De-Distressing

A number of REBT methods lead to solving distress. This includes helping you not only feel much better and get over some of your symptoms, but also make yourself less prone to becoming disturbed over daily matters. With practice, you should rarely become seriously distressed about *anything*.

Unconditional Positive Regard

Also important to mental health is *unconditional positive regard*, or the ability to accept others no matter what they do or how they act or fail. By always avoiding rating a person's self, and instead rating *deeds*, *traits*, and *acts*, you can learn patience.

Higher Frustration Tolerance

Using the principles of REBT, you can raise your frustration tolerance. You can convince yourself that you usually don't *need* what you *want*, that you can stand losses and rejections, and that frustration may be vexatious and aggravating, but that it's never awful, horrible, or utterly bad.

Real-Life Practice

Ellis generally recommends real-life, activity-oriented practice, often referred to as homework assignments, to help you improve your ability to handle difficult situations. You're encouraged to stay with, or endure, frustrating situations (for example, the perception of having a long-term health problem) so that you can learn to tolerate unpleasantness. I'll have more to say about these useful assignments and their application to health anxiety syndrome in chapter 5.

Conclusions

In the end, what probably bothers disease phobics the most is their uncertainty about the physical sensations they experience. Are the sensations normal? What's causing them? Are they the first sign of a serious, deadly disease? As one patient said,

> *The horrible part is never knowing what's wrong. And it surely doesn't help when, after lots of visits to medical doctors and lots of money spent, you still don't have any answers.*

What's the best means of dealing with such doubt? *Don't let your health worries take control!* Instead, try accepting physical frailties and discomforts for what they are—part of being human and alive! We live in a fallible world. Why demand that life be free of hassle and pain? Work at becoming more sensible, and decide to go about your work and life with a more realistic and relaxed attitude about it all.

Now that we've considered the theories behind CBT, let's take a look at some practical applications of self-help therapy for health anxiety syndrome.

Feature: The Perils of Perfectionism

No discussion of cognitive distortions would be complete without a mention of the personality trait of *perfectionism*, which is the irrational pursuit of order, control, flawlessness, faultlessness, precision, exactness, and impeccability. And central to perfectionism is an *obsessive worry* about controlling events—a tendency the person who experiences health anxiety syndrome knows all too well.

From the viewpoint of Allan Mallinger's and Jeannette DeWyze's (1992) book, *Too Perfect: When Being in Control Gets Out of Control*, perfectionism and obsessive worry can lead to health anxieties:

> The wasteland wrought by worry is familiar territory to most obsessives. By worry, I mean thinking repetitively about a current or future problem *in a way that doesn't eventually lead to a solution*. Worry is unproductive by definition, and it seems to have a life of its own.
>
> Almost everyone worries at least occasionally, and this is normal. . . . But many obsessives worry chronically. At times, specific worries fill their consciousness; at other times, worry takes the form of a vague but foreboding presence that subtly drags the worrier down even as he or she goes about the various tasks of daily life. . . .
>
> As if worrying weren't painful enough, the tendency to think in all-or-nothing terms leads many obsessives to envision the very worst outcome possible for their concerns. Marcia, a twenty-nine-year-old music critic, described this very common experience:
>
> "If I notice a strange blemish on my skin, I immediately think, 'What if it's cancer?' And I'm filled with all the dread and horror I would feel if I had already received the diagnosis, and part of my mind is racing ahead, wondering about cancer surgery, thinking about just how painful death from skin cancer is." (pp. 132–134)

To this, Martin Antony and Richard Swinson (1998) added in their book, *When Perfect Isn't Good Enough: Strategies for Coping with Perfectionism*:

> Sometimes health can be the focus of perfectionistic behavior. Some people become very rigid about what they do, for fear of compromising their health. This may include being very particular about foods eaten (e.g., never eating anything containing fat), compulsively exercising, or avoiding computer screens and other devices that give off radiation. Health-obsessed perfectionists may visit doctors frequently to check out unusual symptoms or to have unnecessary medical tests administered. Perfectionism can also cause some people to wash themselves excessively or to avoid touching anything that might be viewed as contaminated (e.g., toilet seats, money, people's hands, etc.). (pp. 16–17)

Question for Thought: How has perfectionism played a part in your own health anxieties?

4

Rethinking Away Your
Health Worries

Irrationally held truths may be more harmful than reasoned errors.

—Thomas Henry Huxley

Now that you understand one of the primary causes of health anxiety syndrome—cognitive distortions—let's see exactly what you can do to solve your health worries. In this chapter, you'll learn how to dispute your irrationalities, replace them with realistic thoughts and self-talk, and practice "thought stopping."

Eliminate Health Anxiety— Starting Today!

Clearly, if you suffer from health anxiety syndrome, your goals are:

- To become more reasonable about health matters

- To find peace within yourself

This is where CBT can prove helpful; it gives you a way to look for those distorted beliefs that are keeping you miserable. And when you challenge your negativities, you show you're committed to keeping a rational attitude about it all.

At the same time, I want to warn you against engaging in *overly* positively thinking. Although it may seem to be affirming (and even "warm and fuzzy"), false positive thinking is irrational in its own right. Consider what Arnold Lazarus and Clifford Lazarus (1997), authors of *The 60-Second Shrink: 101 Strategies for Staying Sane in a Crazy World*, had to say on this topic:

> But there is a big difference between healthy optimism and the Pollyanna pop psychology version of positive thinking. Giddy positivism advises us to look on the bright side at all times. These trite pep talks often tend to backfire and cause resentment and isolation in others.
> People who play the "everything-will-be-terrific" game not only overlook real problems and issues that need to be addressed, but they prevent others from expressing grief, pain, anger, loneliness, or fears. It is difficult if not impossible to air your true feelings in the presence of one of these ever-positive thinkers. They often make others feel guilty for harboring bad feelings. (p. 31)

In other words, this false sense of positive thinking isn't rationality. It's its own cognitive distortion!

Now let's turn our attention to the tools you'll use to change, or reframe, life's problems by modifying your thoughts.

Challenging Your Cognitive Distortions

To overcome your nonsensical thinking, you must first accept the fact that you're a *fallible human being*. By embracing your humanity, you lay the foundation for overcoming your useless worries about illness, disease, pain, and death. After you've done this, you're ready to take steps to eliminate your irrational beliefs.

In the process, you quit *demanding* and *complaining* about not getting what you want. You let go of the *shoulds, oughts, musts,* and *needs*. Only then can you adopt a more realistic perspective of *accepting* and *preferring*.

You take away the *horribleness* and *terribleness* from whatever aspects of life bother you, and acknowledge that nothing is, in fact, ever more than *unfortunate* or *inconvenient*.

Finally, you admit that sicknesses, problems, conflicts, and upsets are, in fact, wonderful opportunities for personal growth, not defeat! In other words, you take control of your thinking and *you decide that you can tolerate virtually anything*.

So, what exactly are the steps in the process of challenging and eliminating irrationalities? Briefly, they are: *identifying* and *considering* your unsound beliefs, *disputing* and *challenging* those beliefs, and *replacing* them with new, sound beliefs. Disputes often look like this:

- "Where is the rule that says . . . ?"

- "What proof do I have that . . . ?"

- "Who says . . . ?"

- "Who cares if . . . ?"

- "What is the probability that . . . ?"

- "What is the worst thing that would happen if . . . ?"

- "Why do I need to . . . ?"

- "So what if . . . ?"

Today's world has certainly provided us with many opportunities to achieve optimal health—at least in theory. But with every hope come letdowns. Sometimes our bodies just won't do what we want them to do. If you've ever been on a diet and tried to shed that last five pounds when you *absolutely, positively,* and *without a doubt* need to lose *immediate* weight to fit into a particular outfit, then you know what I mean.

Here are some cognitive distortions and disputes for a typical person who lets herself get really agitated, for example, when she can't fall sleep:

- "Nothing must interfere with my sleep, because that will be disastrous, and I'll feel miserable and hate life in general."

- "I must be able to fall asleep easily whenever and wherever I wish; otherwise, life is unbearable and I can't be happy at all."

- "It's horrible if I don't get enough sleep. My feeling sleepy during the day is intolerable."

- "My health is certainly in danger if I miss some sleep. The situation is catastrophic; I might get sick or even die as a result of my insomnia."

- "My self-esteem is completely tied up in my ability to control my body. If it doesn't work flawlessly, then I'm automatically inadequate and worthless."

And now for some sample disputes and sensible answers to these irrationalities:

- "Where is the law that says my sleep must never be disturbed?"

- "It's inconvenient if I can't get what I want or fall asleep when I want, but it certainly isn't terrible. I can stand it, just as I've done many times in the past. No matter how poorly I sleep, I can still keep my cool."

- "Sometimes life stinks! But there's no reason for me to get upset about it. Tomorrow always brings new opportunities."

- "Where's the proof that my health is in danger if I miss some sleep? The situation might be uncomfortable, but no one has ever died from insomnia."

- "My self-worth isn't dependent on my mastery of anything. It might be nice if I get enough sleep, but I'm certainly not inadequate or worthless if I don't."

See how it works? Let's try a few more reframes. To get rid of those nonsensical ideas involving your *having* to enjoy radiant health, or the *terribleness* of losing your self-respect if you can't find freedom from chronic pain, follow this simple procedure.

1. First, you identify your *distorted beliefs*, such as:

   • "I *must* enjoy glowing health at all times."

   • "I *must* receive undivided attention from others when I'm sick."

   • "I *must* always be 100 percent in control of my body."

2. Next, consider how your demanding *musts* inevitably lead to *catastrophizing*:

   • "If I don't enjoy glowing health at all times, things are horrible."

   • "If I don't receive undivided attention from others when I'm sick, life is unendurable."

   • "If I don't always have 100 percent control over my body, then I'm a failure and an awful person."

   . . . and how those demands lead to the experience of *low frustration tolerance*:

   • "If life is horrible and I'm a failure and a goof as a person, then I won't be able to stand it."

3. Third, devise *disputes* that rationally challenge your ridiculous thinking:

   • "So what? What's so horrible about that?"

   • "If I don't receive undivided attention from others when I'm sick, why should life be unendurable?"

   • "Where is the proof that if I don't always have 100 percent control over my body, then I'm a failure and an awful person?"

4. And finally, come up with some *sensible replies* to your disputes:

   • "It's inconvenient if I don't enjoy glowing health at all times, but it isn't horrible."

   • "It's uncomfortable when I don't receive the attention I want, but that doesn't mean I can't endure it."

- "It's unfortunate if I can't control my body, but there isn't any rule that says I'm a failure or an awful person because of this."

From these sample distorted beliefs, disputes, and sensible answers, we see that seemingly devastating predicaments aren't necessarily so when facts are separated from illogical assumptions and fears.

Additionally, this CBT approach to health anxiety involves helping you see that it's in your best interest to experience *short-term pain* for the eventual benefits of *long-term gain*. You need to compare the advantages and disadvantages of tolerating momentary discomfort for the sake of future improvement. Increasing tolerance for frustration involves learning to challenge such debilitating thoughts as, "I mustn't experience physical symptoms or discomfort! It's terrible if I do! I can't stand it!" while at the same time developing a more accepting attitude toward bodily ailments in general as part of the human experience.

Practical Pointer

The essential cognitive reframing process can be summarized in these four steps:

1. Identify your cognitive distortions.

2. Consider how your cognitive distortions reflect your tendency to make demands and contribute to your tendency to catastrophize.

3. Devise disputes to challenge your cognitive distortions.

4. Create sensible replies to your disputes.

Thought Stopping

An effective behavioral technique to help you stop worrying about your health is *thought stopping*, which works especially well with the cognitive methods outlined above. This method involves using a physical or verbal trigger to halt an undesirable thought. The trigger can be an action such as clapping your hands or snapping your fingers, or something you say to yourself out loud, such as the word

STOP. (In chapter 5, you'll find more ideas for triggers you can use.) The trigger, whatever it may be, forces a clean break from the unproductive, disabling thought and paves the way for more practical thinking.

Once you become more aware of your irrational self-talk, you can begin editing and controlling your internal voice to feed you with confidence-enhancing, sensible statements instead of critical, anxious, and guilt-producing ones. You'll want to make a deliberate effort to eliminate disabling thoughts and build on your best thoughts and emotions.

In short, first identify and challenge any irrational beliefs or unrealistic expectations. Then use thought stopping.

Let's try one:

Cognitive Distortion: "Oh no, I've got a rash on my foot again. That means they'll probably have to amputate my . . ."
Thought Stopping: "STOP!"

Or this one:

Cognitive Distortion: "I just know I caught AIDS when that condom broke. I bet I only have six months to live before . . ."
Thought Stopping: "STOP!"

Easy, isn't it? It's also very effective in stopping irrational thoughts! And it works even better if you take some time for intentional relaxation immediately after using the technique.

Thought stopping is helpful when you have toxic thoughts that keep you from finding happiness, good health, and peace of mind. You should use thought stopping whenever you find yourself focusing on unwanted thoughts. Rest assured that as you continue to use this method, you'll discover how to take control of your cognitive distortions. The frequency of these thoughts will lessen with time.

Finally, before trying this behavioral technique, you must admit that *your health anxieties are of your own making.* No one "out there" is forcing you to obsess over your health.

Practice Makes Perfect?

Of course, psychological techniques like the ones just described are only techniques. To find true and lasting calmness of mind, you'll probably have to work hard at changing your irrational thinking patterns. This means you'll want to *practice, practice, practice!* (But don't worry about perfection!) Why? Because when you practice a new activity, you effectively train it into your nervous system. I'm

Practical Pointer

Identify cognitive distortions and practice thought stopping whenever they occur. As soon as you notice irrational self-talk, loudly say "STOP" to help clear your mind. Then turn your attention to something more rational. If you still can't stop thinking about your health, try distracting yourself. Exercise. Read a book. Watch a movie. Focus your attention on something or someone else.

sure you've learned to type on a keyboard or play a musical instrument. When you first begin to master a new skill, it all seems rather awkward. Your hands don't want to do what your head tells them to do. Every motion requires considerable conscious thought and effort to execute, and you can quickly become discouraged. Nevertheless, after many, many hours of practice, the new skill becomes more automatic, so that you no longer need to concentrate so intensely.

The same is true of learning and mastering the cognitive reframing techniques described in this chapter. Once you've practiced and trained your nervous system into accepting this approach, you won't have to think about the techniques in order to use them. They'll become an instinctive reflex, available whenever you need them.

In his book entitled *Don't Believe It for a Minute! Forty Toxic Ideas That Are Driving You Crazy*, Arnold Lazarus (1993) described it this way:

> One good rule of thumb: every time you catch yourself thinking a toxic or negative thought, make yourself consider at least two (more is better) positive self-statements or healthy counter-beliefs. This will help you work toward increasing psychological balance. At first this mental exercise might seem unnatural, but after a little practice, you will feel an increasing sense of familiarity with positive thoughts, making it progressively easier to achieve a more balanced mind and a winning and loving lifestyle. (p. 6)

At the end of this chapter is a Cognitive Reframing Chart to help you practice identifying and challenging the irrationalities in your life. Photocopy the chart, and whenever you recognize a personal cognitive distortion, record it and the situation in which it occurred. Then write your disputes and sensible replies. Also, try rating your level of distress both before and after you apply cognitive restructuring to your irrational thinking. Here's what a sample entry might look like:

Situation: Experiencing heartburn or indigestion following a large meal.
Rating of Distress Prior to Cognitive Reframing (1 = least distress to 5 = most distress): 5
Cognitive Distortion: "I must have cancer of the esophagus."
Dispute: "What's the likelihood that I have cancer of the esophagus?"
Sensible Reply: "While it's possible that I have cancer of the esophagus, it's not probable."
Rating of Distress Following Cognitive Reframing (1 = least distress to 5 = most distress): 2

Get the idea? Here's another scenario:

Situation: Fear over the results of an upcoming blood test.
Rating of Distress Prior to Cognitive Reframing (1 = least distress to 5 = most distress): 5
Cognitive Distortion: "Oh no, I'm just sure tomorrow's blood test will reveal very bad news. I'll probably be diagnosed with diabetes."
Dispute: "What's so catastrophic about receiving bad news?"
Sensible Reply: "Even if I do receive bad news, I can handle it. Having a disease or condition is inconvenient, but it's perfectly tolerable."
Rating of Distress Following Cognitive Reframing (1 = least distress to 5 = most distress): 1

When you use this charting method, besides getting practice at cognitive reframing, you might also discover some unhealthy patterns in other areas of your life that could also use some improvement.

Situation: Fear of possibly handling contaminated mail.
Rating of Distress Prior to Cognitive Reframing (1 = least distress to 5 = most distress): 5
Cognitive Distortion: "I just know I'm going to contact inhalation anthrax from opening my mail."
Dispute: "How likely is it that I'll contact an anthrax infection?"
Sensible Reply: "It's possible that I might contract inhalation anthrax, but it's very improbable."
Rating of Distress Following Cognitive Reframing (1 = least distress to 5 = most distress): 3

Keeping Track of It All

Most of my clients find it useful to keep track of their practice sessions on paper (you might try using the Cognitive Reframing Chart at the end of the chapter). With practice, though, you'll find it becomes easier and easier to dispute nonsensical thinking in your head without having to write anything down. For instance, you might catch yourself worrying about a wart on your back. But instead of calling 911, you'll automatically relax and remind yourself that there's no evidence the wart is life-threatening.

Here's a brief excerpt from a counseling session in which I verbally guided a client through the cognitive restructuring process—similar to what you can do either in your head or on paper.

Jill: I'm really worried that I'm going to get uterine cancer and need a hysterectomy.

Dr. Z: So, you're worried about getting cancer and needing a hysterectomy?

Jill: Yes, that's it.

Dr. Z: Any reason to believe any of this is going to happen?

Jill: I'm not sure. I just have this funny feeling.

Dr. Z: Have you had a physical exam from a doctor?

Jill: Yes, and she assured me that everything is fine.

Dr. Z: Do you have a family history of uterine cancer?

Jill: No, no family history. But I get cramps every now and then.

Dr. Z: How often?

Jill: About once a month . . . during my period.

Dr. Z: You think you're going to get cancer because you have occasional cramps?

Jill: That's right.

Dr. Z: Jill, given what we've talked about . . . you know, irrational beliefs and the like, do you maybe see a fallacy in your thinking?

Jill: Well . . .

Dr. Z: Let's look at it this way. Where's the evidence that having menstrual cramps means an automatic diagnosis of uterine cancer?

Jill: I guess there isn't any. But I still worry about it. I can't bear the thought of having an illness like that.

Dr. Z: You're *demanding* to have perfect health; otherwise, you can't stand it? Is that it?

Jill: Yes.

Dr. Z: You *require* that your health be what you want it to be?

Jill: Yes.

Dr. Z: And *you're telling yourself* that to experience discomfort, in your case cramps, is totally bad. And if it's totally bad, then it means disease and death.

Jill: Well, yes, but that's starting to sound silly.

Dr. Z: Why?

Jill: I guess because I'm catastrophizing about my cramps.

Dr. Z: Exactly. Where's your proof that cancer is looming in your future?

Jill: I don't have any.

Dr. Z: And what's the probability that your cramps are a sign of cancer?

Jill: I suppose very little.

Dr. Z: Bravo! What does this mean for you?

Jill: That I can relax and not worry about it. But it's so hard.

Dr. Z: Of course. But you *can* quit worrying. You just need to set your mind to it and practice the techniques that we've been talking about these past couple of weeks.

After taking yourself through a mental routine like this session or filling out the Cognitive Reframing Chart, you'll be cured, right? It'd be nice if life were that simple and straightforward, but it isn't. Cognitive therapy takes time, motivation, and self-reflection, but the rewards of rationality and peace of mind are definitely worth the time and effort spent.

Conclusions

Cognitive behavioral therapy uses a combination of cognitive, emotive, and behavioral techniques to reveal your deepest irrational and self-destructive philosophies. It also offers tools to help you modify these. The goal in CBT, including REBT, is to help you accept reality, surrender your demands and compulsivity, and maximize your freedom of choice to find answers to your problems.

Don't get me wrong, though. None of the above is easy to carry out. Changing long-term, deeply embedded patterns is *tough*, but it can be done with motivation and perseverance on your part. Only *you* have the power to let go of those health worries. Only *you* can make it all happen!

In the next chapter, I present several other psychological and medical methods used to treat health anxiety syndrome, particularly in those cases requiring the expertise of a licensed professional.

Feature: Handling Guilt, Depression, and Anger

As I've already mentioned, once you realize nothing is actually wrong with you (following numerous medical appointments and tests, all of which confirm nothing), you'll probably experience some serious embarrassment over your fears. You might think you've made a fool of yourself in front of your doctor, family, friends, and coworkers. You might feel guilty about having inconvenienced your loved ones. Or you might feel terribly angry at yourself for having given into irrational thinking about your health.

If any of this rings true for you, you've probably learned some irrational self-talk about health and emotions, such as:

- "Nice people don't act or think like that."

- "Shame on you for getting sick!"

- "Good people take care of themselves and stay healthy."

- "You must never complain or bother anybody."

- "You must never lose your temper."

This irrational self-talk has probably prompted you to believe such cognitive distortions as:

- "I don't always act or think like a nice person, so I must be a lousy person."

- "I occasionally fall ill, so I must be a shame to everyone around me and a moral disaster."

- "Sometimes I complain, so that means I'm a worthless person who wants to upset everyone."

- "I get mad sometimes, so that means I'm a failure."

Of course, such self-talk isn't exclusive to disease phobics. You'll find it's common among lots of people with different kinds of problems. I'm confident you, too, can relate to at least a few of the above, and probably come up with more of your own.

It might sound like I believe guilt, depression, and anger are necessarily bad. Quite to the contrary. Like so many aspects of life, these emotional states have both positive and negative sides—specifically, both *constructive* (rational) and *destructive* (irrational) sides. Constructive emotions (for example, depression in response to the loss of a loved one) are present-focused and healthy expressions of normal psychological processes; they help you process events and move on. In contrast, destructive emotions (including chronic hostility or grudges over injustices experienced long ago) are past-focused and self-defeating; they keep you trapped in the past so that you can't make effective decisions in the present. You become so focused on yesterday's irritations or mistakes that you're blinded to today's joys.

Where do these destructive emotions come from? What's behind all the negativity? Essentially, the guilt, depression, and anger that we're talking about are but additional examples of absolutistic, irrational thinking. Unlike anxiety's *what ifs* (which are often future-focused), guilt has as its core various *if onlys* (which are often past-focused). For instance:

- "*If only* I had lived up to my potential!"

- "*If only* I hadn't lost my temper at my husband!"

- "*If only* I had taken better care of myself!"

- "*If only* people had treated me better when I was young!"

. . . which translate into:

- "I *should* have lived up to my potential!"

- "I *should* have loved my husband more!"

- "I *should* have taken better care of myself!"

- "People *should* have treated me better when I was young!"

. . . which all imply:

- "I'm a valueless person for failing to do or be what I *should* do or be, or *should* have done or been."

- "I *must* find the ideal solution to yesterday's problems."

- "My past *must* determine how I think and what I do in the present, and continue to do so forever."

We see from these sample cognitive distortions that irrational emotions begin with arbitrary *if onlys*, move to *shoulds* and *musts,* and end with finger pointing and self-loathing. This is because irrational emotions are strong motivators, but they're the wrong kind of motivators. Instead of encouraging personal growth, they push us into desperate attempts to live up to someone else's expectations and standards. And, of course, we know what happens when you try to do that. You *blunder.* And when you blunder, you feel like a *failure*, you become *depressed.* And when you become depressed, you *berate* and *blame* yourself. And when you berate and blame yourself, you feel *guilty* for being imperfect and fallible—all of which sets the stage for you to feel *angry* at yourself, others, and the world. Put simply, you get caught in a never-ending, self-defeating cycle that fuels itself every time you give in to nonsensical thinking, talking, and doing.

Can anything be done about destructive emotions? In addition to the cognitive reframing techniques presented in

Stop Worrying About Your Health!, there's another strategy that can help you: *acceptance*. In striving to improve our lives, we *accept* our limitations and imperfections. We *accept* that we're going to make mistakes. We *accept* that others aren't always going to treat us fairly. We *accept* that life isn't always going to give us what we want when we want it. Embracing acceptance in this way eliminates negativity, and leads us to be assertive and enjoy a rewarding and productive life.

Have the courage to admit that you're a fallible human being and then *forgive yourself and others* for all sins, deficiencies, mistakes, inadequacies, faults, and shortcomings. As I mentioned earlier, accepting your imperfect nature is crucial to attaining emotional health and freedom from your physical symptoms.

Questions for Thought: Which emotion has bothered you the most: guilt, depression, or anger? Why do you think that is?

Cognitive Reframing Chart

You can create a chart like this in a notebook or on individual sheets of paper. Just be sure to give yourself plenty of space to write.

1. Situation:

Rating of Distress Prior to Cognitive Reframing (1 = least distress to
    5 = most distress):
Cognitive Distortion:
Dispute:
Sensible Reply:
Rating of Distress Following Cognitive Reframing (1 = least distress
    to 5 = most distress):

2. Situation:

Rating of Distress Prior to Cognitive Reframing (1 = least distress to
    5 = most distress):
Cognitive Distortion:
Dispute:
Sensible Reply:
Rating of Distress Following Cognitive Reframing (1 = least distress
    to 5 = most distress):

3. Situation:

Rating of Distress Prior to Cognitive Reframing (1 = least distress to
    5 = most distress):
Cognitive Distortion:
Dispute:
Sensible Reply:
Rating of Distress Following Cognitive Reframing (1 = least distress
    to 5 = most distress):

4. Situation:

Rating of Distress Prior to Cognitive Reframing (1 = least distress to
    5 = most distress):
Cognitive Distortion:
Dispute:
Sensible Reply:
Rating of Distress Following Cognitive Reframing (1 = least distress
    to 5 = most distress):

5. Situation:

Rating of Distress Prior to Cognitive Reframing (1 = least distress to
    5 = most distress):
Cognitive Distortion:
Dispute:
Sensible Reply:
Rating of Distress Following Cognitive Reframing (1 = least distress
    to 5 = most distress):

6. Situation:

Rating of Distress Prior to Cognitive Reframing (1 = least distress to
    5 = most distress):
Cognitive Distortion:
Dispute:
Sensible Reply:
Rating of Distress Following Cognitive Reframing (1 = least distress
    to 5 = most distress):

7. Situation:

Rating of Distress Prior to Cognitive Reframing (1 = least distress to
    5 = most distress):
Cognitive Distortion:
Dispute:
Sensible Reply:
Rating of Distress Following Cognitive Reframing (1 = least distress
    to 5 = most distress):

8. Situation:

Rating of Distress Prior to Cognitive Reframing (1 = least distress to
    5 = most distress):
Cognitive Distortion:
Dispute:
Sensible Reply:
Rating of Distress Following Cognitive Reframing (1 = least distress
    to 5 = most distress):

5

Medical and Behavioral Approaches to Health Anxiety Syndrome

Attention to health is the greatest hindrance to life.

—Plato

In this chapter, we'll review some of the standard psychological and medical and behavioral therapies for health anxieties, with a focus on current methods that have been shown to be effective for the greatest number of people.

According to most of the clinical literature, the usual goal of treatment is to help people with health anxiety (and their families) live with their symptoms while *changing* the thinking patterns and behavior that reinforce and perpetuate their unwanted physical symptoms and anxieties. We talked at length about this approach in the previous two chapters, which hopefully made the case that supportive cognitive behavioral therapies (such as REBT and Beck's model) are quite effective for eliminating this problem.

One example of a psychological model that doesn't seem to help people with health anxiety syndrome much is long-term insight-oriented treatment (for example, Freudian psychoanalysis and psychodynamic therapy). Why? Because most disease phobics resist the childhood-focused psychological interpretations characteristic of Freudian models, so they often end up prematurely dropping out of these forms of therapy when they don't experience results. If you have health anxiety, you're probably more likely to benefit from the cognitive methods outlined already, as well as from the behavioral methods—relaxation training, visualization, distraction techniques, hypnosis, biofeedback, and more—that I describe in this chapter.

Medical Techniques

Before reviewing an assortment of behavioral techniques available for helping you overcome your worries, let's take a quick look at a typical medical approach to treating health anxiety.

Without a doubt, if you experience health anxiety syndrome, you've probably spent a great deal of time in medical offices, emergency rooms, hospitals, and clinics. This makes sense, because you've tried over and over to get to the bottom of your bodily problems, but to no avail. It's logical to assume that medical problems need medical solutions. But, ironically, this isn't the case with health anxiety syndrome. Medical treatment—which usually consists of medications (such as antidepressants and tranquilizers) or, in more extreme cases, surgery—is perhaps the worst approach to take with health anxiety, even though your common sense might dictate otherwise. While the use of medications to relieve anxiety and depression is possible in some instances, this approach hasn't been shown to *solve* the problem of health anxiety; it only temporarily bandages your wounds.

In my experience with health anxiety clients, I've noticed a fascinating pattern. The physical symptoms might temporarily improve following standard medical treatment, but they frequently return or move to another part of the body. And this is why medical treatment often proves fruitless. *You can't effectively treat a psychological problem in the same manner that you treat a physical problem.* We've shown in previous chapters that, while health anxiety syndrome definitely has a physical component and can even coexist or be triggered by bodily illnesses, the problem is essentially caused by irrational thinking patterns about physical symptoms, health status, illness, disease, discomfort, and so on. Because the cause is primarily mental, the cure must also be primarily mental. In the long run, doctor shopping, seeking unnecessary medical testing, trying a myriad of medications, having surgeries, overexercising, and overcontrolling your diet probably aren't going to eliminate your physical symptoms or relieve your health anxieties.

Practical Pointer

You can't effectively treat a psychological problem in the same manner that you treat a physical problem.

As I've already mentioned in *Stop Worrying About Your Health!*, if you're troubled by physical symptoms, you do need to see a health-care professional to rule out the presence of a physical disorder. But after you've had all the necessary medical tests, sought a second opinion, and been repeatedly assured there's nothing wrong with you physically, it's definitely time to begin *rethinking* how you look at life, including your health.

Practical Pointer

If you have physical symptoms, you need to see a health-care professional to rule out the presence of a physical disorder. But after you've been repeatedly assured there's nothing wrong, it's definitely time to begin rethinking *how you look at life.*

Cognitive Techniques
First and Foremost!

In the last chapter, I explained how cognitive techniques like rational-emotive-behavior therapy (REBT) can be so important for self-managing health anxiety syndrome. Let's briefly review how these methods works.

In a nutshell, you decide when and under what conditions your thinking process has become dysfunctional. Once you've identified the source of your problematic thinking, it's time to dispute and alter your perspectives in a way that creates non-problematic thinking. Then, after a time of effective practice (sometimes within hours), the problem or discomfort is often eliminated. In other words, *by altering your irrational perceptions and replacing them with rational ones, it becomes possible to recondition your mind to operate in new, healthier ways.* As a reminder, the process goes like this:

1. Use the Cognitive Reframing Chart found at the end of chapter 4.

2. Identify your cognitive distortions.

3. Dispute and challenge your cognitive distortions.

4. Replace your cognitive distortions with sensible thoughts.

5. *Practice, practice, and practice!*

In my professional opinion and experience, this straightforward cognitive approach to health anxiety syndrome is the most effective for the most people. *Cognitive therapy is your first, best hope for overcoming health anxiety syndrome.* And while such psychological treatments as "insight therapies" (long-term process-oriented therapies, like psychodynamic counseling and psychoanalysis) might have value in certain cases of disease phobias, I don't tend to recommend them. However, I do recommend a number of behavioral therapies to help you retrain your mind by changing your behavior.

Behavioral Techniques

As I indicated in chapter 2, the *behavioral perspective* holds that most, if not all, mental functioning is directly related to behavior and learning. Thus, *behaviorists*—clinicians who primarily use behavioral techniques to treat problems—are concerned with the roles that behavior and learning play in life. They base their views on *learning theory*, which is a body of psychological theories proposing that modifications in behavior occur as a result of experience. Since the 1950s, many psychological problems (for example, smoking, overeating) have been shown to respond favorably to treatment with behavior therapy.

Several of the more popular behavioral therapies that can be used to treat health worries include *systematic desensitization* (which includes *behavioral analysis*, *relaxation training*, and developing a *graduated hierarchy*), *modeling therapy*, *exposure and response therapy*, *thought stopping and distraction*, *stress management*, *imagery and visualization*, *hypnosis*, *biofeedback*, and *homework assignments*. Not surprisingly, you can't perform most behavioral therapies without scheduling at least a few sessions with a licensed clinician. However, I want to give a brief overview of these methods in the event you decide to seek professional help for your health anxieties.

Systematic Desensitization

Whenever a pattern of cognitive, emotional, or physical behavior is maladaptive (interferes with successful functioning in your personal or social environment) and is also considered a phobia or anxiety disorder, the behavioral treatment of choice is *systematic desensitization*, also known as *graduated exposure*. Although the psychological literature generally recommends systematic desensitization to treat irrational fears, phobias, and anxieties, this behavioral technique has also been shown to be helpful for treating a wide range of other problems, including alcoholism, drug abuse, depression, sexual dysfunctions, tension headaches, muscle tension, asthma, hyperacidity of the stomach, and hypertension.

Joseph Wolpe developed systematic desensitization when he became disenchanted with traditional psychoanalytical treatments (Wolpe 1958). Serving in the South African Medical Corps during World War II, Wolpe discovered that an emphasis on exploring childhood memories and using Freudian "free association" was ineffective for treating soldiers with "war neurosis." Wolpe believed that his patients needed to be "deconditioned" because of their *learned* anxiety in association with traumatic situations. He then began to research and empirically test his theory, and later developed this powerful behavioral treatment.

The procedure of systematic desensitization consists of three basic parts: 1) a complete *behavioral analysis* of the client's situation, 2) *relaxation training*, and 3) *hierarchy construction* and *presentation*.

Behavioral analysis. This involves a complete psychological evaluation based on self-reports of behavior. In other words, behavioral analysis involves a therapist asking you about your anxiety and fears, specifically in terms of how you respond to certain stimuli. If your fear or anxiety disrupts your ability to function successfully in the world, systematic desensitization might then be indicated as a treatment possibility.

Relaxation training. When confronted with stressful situations, we often prepare ourselves to run or fight. This "fight or flight" response helps our bodies to reach a state of emergency-level readiness. If you've ever accidentally stepped off of a curb only to be almost hit by a car, you've probably noticed that your heart and breathing rates instantly and automatically increase. This is the fight or flight response in action; it's there to protect you—in this case, making you jump out of the way of the car. So, when you're in real, immediate danger, it's appropriate to feel afraid. Getting your body revved up with adrenaline could very well keep you alive.

The problem comes, though, when we don't need this level of readiness—when running or fighting isn't required. In other words, most of the time when we feel stressed, there's no imminent danger, so it's a false alarm. Put simply, the fire alarm is ringing, but there isn't a fire!

When the fight or flight response activates in the absence of a threatening situation, we typically experience anxiety or panic. Our modern-day lives keep us so busy that we're often too wound up. If our bodies remain in this heightened state for long periods of time, in addition to anxiety we can develop such bodily symptoms as headaches, tension, back pain, or stomach trouble. *No doubt, at least some of the experience and symptoms of health anxiety are due to chronic high levels of stress.* (Refer back to chapter 2 for more information on the role of stress in mind-body problems.)

Practical Pointer

If you remain in a "high gear" state for long periods of time, besides anxiety you can develop such symptoms as headaches, tension, back pain, or stomach trouble. At least some of the experience and symptoms of health anxiety are due to chronic high levels of stress.

Many methods are available for learning to cope better with stress. One is to learn relaxation techniques, which can help lessen the degree of unproductive physical arousal that most of us experience these days.

Applied relaxation is now considered an established and efficient psychological therapy for anxiety, phobias, and panic. In many cases, applied relaxation is just as effective as other behavioral methods, and it brings about significant improvements in nearly all cases.

Once your therapist determines that systematic desensitization is appropriate for you, you're taught techniques of *progressive muscle relaxation* (PMR), which involves the sequential contracting and relaxing of muscles. The goal is to assist you in achieving a feeling of muscular and mental relaxation. You start by relaxing your forehead and facial muscles—tensing these groups for a few seconds and then relaxing them. Next, you move down your body from your neck and shoulders to your shoulder blades, upper back, arms, hands, lower back, legs, and feet. You can also practice deep breathing during PMR by inhaling when you tense your muscles and then exhaling when you relax them.

Although you learn PMR in your therapist's office, you should also practice it between sessions until you feel competent. You might also learn to use SUDS (subjective units of distress scale), in which you assign a numerical score ranging from 0 to 100 to the degree of anxiety you feel. The more anxiety or tension you experience, the higher will be your SUDS score. As you learn to relax, you should see your SUDS diminish.

Setting aside time to relax and get yourself "centered" can be of immense value in managing health anxiety syndrome. Here are two of my favorite, quick (about ten minutes each) relaxation procedures. The first is found in Sharon Johnson's (1997) *Therapist's Guide to Clinical Intervention*:

- Get comfortable.

- You are going to count backwards from ten to zero.

- Silently say each number as you exhale.

- As you count, you will relax more deeply and go deeper and deeper into a state of relaxation.

- When you reach zero, you will be completely relaxed.

- You feel more and more relaxed, you can feel the tension leave your body.

- You are becoming as limp as a rag doll; the tension is going away.

- You are very relaxed.

- Now drift deeper with each breath, deeper and deeper.

- Feel the deep relaxation all over and continue relaxing.

- Now, relaxing deeper, you should feel an emotional calm.

- Tranquil and serene feelings, feelings of safety and security, and a calm peace.

- Try to get a quiet inner confidence.

- Get a good feeling about yourself and relaxation.

- Study once more the feelings that come with relaxation.

- Let your muscles switch off; feel good about everything.

- Calm and serene surroundings make you feel more and more tranquil and peaceful.

- You will continue to relax for several minutes.

- When I tell you to start, count from one to three, silently saying each number as you take a deep breath.

- Open your eyes when you get to three. You will be relaxed and alert.

- When you open your eyes you will find yourself back in the place where you started your relaxation.

- The environment will seem slower and more calm.

- You will be more relaxed and peaceful.

- Now count from one to three. (p. 153)

Deep breathing exercises are another very easy way to relax your body. Most of us tend to fill only the upper chest when we breathe. We may not even realize that the increased oxygen intake we get from deep breathing can actually relieve tension and improve mental alertness. Just notice how an infant's abdomen rises and falls with each breath. Now that's true deep breathing!

By using one or both of the deep breathing exercises provided below, you can quickly relax, as well as potentially improve your circulation, oxygenate your blood, strengthen your lungs, and relieve various respiratory ailments.

Here is a deep breathing exercise from *The Relaxation and Stress Reduction Workbook* by Martha Davis, Elizabeth Robbins Eshelman, and Matthew McKay (2000).

- Although this exercise can be practiced in a variety of poses, the following is recommended: Lie down on a blanket or rug on the floor. Bend your knees and move your feet about eight inches apart, with your toes turned slightly outward. Make sure that your spine is straight.

- Scan your body for tension.

- Place one hand on your abdomen and one hand on your chest.

- Inhale slowly and deeply through your nose into your abdomen to push up your hand as much as feels comfortable. Your chest should move only a little and only with your abdomen.

- When you feel at ease with the above step, smile slightly and inhale through your nose and exhale through your mouth, making a quiet, relaxing, whooshing sound like the wind as you blow gently out. Your mouth, tongue, and jaw will be relaxed. Take long, slow, deep breaths that raise and lower your abdomen. Focus on the sound and feeling of breathing as you become more and more relaxed.

- Continue deep breathing for about five or ten minutes at a time, once or twice a day. Then, if you like, gradually extend this period to twenty minutes.

- At the end of each deep breathing session, take a little time to once more scan your body for tension. Compare the tension you feel at the conclusion of the exercise with that which you experienced when you began.

- When you become at ease with breathing into your abdomen, practice it at any time during the day when you feel like it and you are sitting down or standing still. Concentrate on your abdomen moving up and down, the air moving in and out of your lungs, and the feeling of relaxation that deep breathing gives you.

- When you have learned to relax yourself using deep breathing, practice it whenever you feel yourself getting tense. (p. 25)

And an even shorter exercise for deep breathing is:

- Sit or lie down in a quiet place where you won't be disturbed for several minutes.

- Recall some good, positive feelings.

- Close your mouth and relax all of your muscles.

- Slowly and deeply inhale through your nose (not your mouth) to a count of six or eight. As you do this, consciously push out your abdomen.

- Hold your breath to a count of four.

- Slowly breathe out through your mouth (not your nose) to a count of six or eight.

- Continue to repeat this "inhale-hold-exhale" cycle until you achieve maximum relaxation.

Still another relaxation method is known as *rapid relaxation*, in which you use anxiety-triggering thoughts as a cue to bring on a brief relaxation state. When you find your anxiety rising, take a couple of deep breaths, say the word *relax*, and exhale. You perform rapid relaxation while mentally scanning your body for tension and trying to relax everything as much as possible.

Graduated hierarchy. The next step in systematic desensitization involves creating a *graduated hierarchy* of your fears, ordered from lowest to highest anxiety-arousing situations. Completion of a hierarchy typically requires three to five sessions, although the process can take as little as one session or as many as twenty-five or more.

The final step in Wolpe's procedure is for the therapist to present the distressing situations in the graduated hierarchy first *covertly* (in the imagination), and then *overtly* (in vivo). Meanwhile, during these "exposure" sessions, you practice PMR in response to each item on your hierarchy. In this way, you move step-by-step up your hierarchy as you become more at ease with whatever it is that frightens you.

For Personal Reflection

Try creating your own health anxiety hierarchy. Below list your top ten health-related fears beginning with the least anxiety-provoking (#10) and ending with the most anxiety-provoking (#1).

1.

2.

3.

4.

5.

6.

7.

8.

9.

10.

What did you learn while completing this exercise?

Let's take a look at some of the specifics of this procedure. First, during the *covert* portion of systematic desensitization, you're asked to relax and to visualize the least distressing item on your hierarchy. If you can imagine the scene without an anxiety response for a minimum of ten seconds, the therapist presents the next item on the list. On the other hand, if you have anxiety, you're directed to stop imagining the scene and tell your therapist about your anxiety. Once you again become relaxed, you return to that item for a shorter period of time. Then you gradually increase your imagery times for that scene until you can easily visualize it twice in a row for at least ten seconds each. You continue this process until you're able to handle comfortably every item on your hierarchy.

Second, during the in vivo portion of systematic desensitization, you learn to transfer, or generalize, your reduced anxiety levels to real-life situations (i.e., the real-life equivalents to your imaginal hierarchy). In vivo practice is extremely important. As you seek out actual counterparts to the imagined scenes, you reinforce in real life what you learned in sessions.

Modeling Therapy

Health anxiety is often treated favorably with *modeling therapy*. In this procedure, you observe someone else (called the *model* or *actor*) approach an anxiety-provoking object or participate in an anxiety-provoking activity that is comparable to your specific problem. The goal in modeling therapy is for you to relearn how to react under similar circumstances.

Practical Pointer

Systematic desensitization is a specific behavioral technique that interrupts the link between anxiety-inducing objects or events and the anxiety response. This treatment requires you to systematically confront the objects of your fear. The three main elements to the process include 1) relaxation training, 2) generating a list that prioritizes anxiety-producing situations by degree of fear, and 3) the desensitization procedure itself, which involves confronting each item on the list beginning with the least stressful. Systematic desensitization is particularly effective for anxiety-related problems, including disease phobias.

Although a live model is probably more effective, you can also watch a videotape of someone engaging in the activity. And if you have access to such technology, a virtual reality session can also be a beneficial modeling tool. This technology uses computer-generated images and special headgear to simulate a realistic social environment that allows you to interact with it.

Exposure and Response Therapy

Unlike systematic desensitization, in which you learn to relax while gradually confronting your anxiety, *exposure and response therapy* intentionally causes anxiety. By repeatedly exposing yourself to a feared situation or object (be it in vivo or covertly), you experience such intense and sustained anxiety that it eventually loses its power over you.

Two types of exposure therapy commonly used in cases of anxiety are *graduated exposure* and *flooding*. Graduated exposure offers you a greater degree of direction over the frequency and length of exposures. Flooding involves your being continuously exposed to anxiety-inducing events—for hours in some cases. Both types of exposure and response therapy begin with the most feared stimulus, unlike systematic desensitization which begins with the least feared stimulus.

Combining exposure with cognitive therapy appears to be very useful for some disease phobics.

Thought Stopping and Distraction

As you become more aware of your tendency to engage in negative self-talk, you'll want to begin editing and controlling your "inner voice" in order to fill your mind with positive, confidence-enhancing self-talk rather than cognitive distortions of anxiety, shame, and self-criticism. You'll have to make a conscious effort to remove your distorted thoughts while building upon the thoughts and feelings that have characterized the happiest, most confident times of your life.

Thought stopping is an excellent means of eliminating negative self-talk. You'll recall from chapter 4 that this technique involves using a verbal or physical trigger to halt undesirable thinking. The most popular trigger is the word *STOP*, said out loud or to yourself. You might even try screaming "STOP" inside your head. You can also clap your hands, snap your fingers, squeeze your eyes tightly shut, think of a large red stop sign, or pop your wrist with a rubber band. Whichever you choose, your trigger allows you to break free from unproductive, debilitating thinking. Remember, you should be consistent in your use of thought stopping; use it every time you have irrational thoughts. As you continue to use this technique, you'll gain control of your thinking and see the frequency of negative self-talk decrease.

Thought distraction involves shifting your thoughts. One method is to think about something that's calming and positive, such as a birthday celebration, a vacation you're planning, or a time when you felt delighted. Another method is to think about complex matters so that your mind becomes completely occupied. Two good examples of thought distraction are saying the alphabet backwards and counting by sevens in your head.

Don't forget that the more you practice these techniques, the better they work. In the beginning, it can be tough to shift your thoughts for more than a few seconds at a time. But with practice, thought stopping and distraction will become second nature to you.

Stress Management

One applied topic of psychology that has received a great deal of attention in recent decades is *stress*, or the internal sense that your resources to cope with demands will soon be depleted. Why has stress been studied so extensively? *Because the higher your stress levels, the more likely you are to develop physical symptoms or an illness.* We can all relate to stress, but the problem does seem to be particularly common among those who experience health anxiety syndrome.

Stress occurs in all age groups, although it seems to be increasingly common as we get older and have to cope with mortgages, career burnout, children, and aging parents. As one example of this, stress is keenly felt in adults who work. The most common sources of stress in the workplace include lack of expected progress (including promotions and raises), lack of creative input into decision-making, lack of challenging work, inadequate pay, monotonous tasks, feelings of being underutilized, vague job descriptions and procedures, conflicts with the boss or supervisor, lack of quality vacation time, workaholism, sexual harassment, forced career changes, and sudden job loss. In addition to an assortment of unpleasant physical symptoms (such as migraines, ulcers, and allergies), long-term job stress can eventually result in *burnout*, a state of mental exhaustion characterized by feelings of helplessness and loss of control, as well as the inability to cope with or complete assigned work.

Resistance to stress, known as *hardiness*, varies from person to person. Hardiness probably results from your adeptness at *cognitive appraisal*, or interpretation of stressors, and the degree to which you feel "in control" of stressors, as well as your personality type, genetics, and lifestyle habits. For the most part, the reasons we become stressed are closely tied to the way we think about what's going on around us. Yes, past experiences can heavily influence us, but the *mechanism* of that influence is our thinking. For instance, if you were neglected as a young child, you might have the erroneous belief that you don't deserve to be happy or loved. In this case, it's today's belief that's bothering you, not the neglect from years ago. The point is that we have a substantial degree of control over ourselves and how we react to our circumstances.

Believe it or not, you can learn how to eliminate a great deal of stress from your life. I don't mean ridding yourself of life's pressures; these are inevitable. Think of it this way: pressure is what happens to you, and stress is your reaction to that pressure. The key to stress management, then, is changing the way you look at pressure—in other words, *cognitive reframing*.

Thankfully, stress management is a skill you can learn. Here are a few simple ways to reduce stress in your life:

- *Learn to relax.* This helps your body learn how to "shut off" the fight or flight response. Relaxation methods (like PMR, described above) are based on the concept that you can't be apprehensive and relaxed at the same time. In essence, whatever you do that opposes the fight or flight response will usually turn it off.

- *Practice deep breathing.* Take slow, deep breaths rather than the fast, shallow ones you probably tend to take during times of stress.

- *Imagine a very peaceful scene,* either a real one or made-up one. Try to involve all of your senses as you imagine this relaxing place.

- *Develop social support.* Keep in mind that people with adequate social support networks report less stress and overall enhanced psychological health in comparison to those without quality social contacts.

- *Avoid stressful situations whenever possible,* and practice the cognitive restructuring techniques that are the basis of *Stop Worrying About Your Health!*

Imagery and Visualization

Imagery, otherwise known as *guided imagery* or *visualization*, is used to change attitudes, behavior, or bodily reactions. It's a well-

Practical Pointer

Keep in mind that the basic premise of cognitive therapy is that our emotions and behaviors are largely influenced by our thinking. The simplest explanation for why cognitive techniques work to eliminate stress is that calming thoughts cause relaxation, which is incompatible with stress. Eliminating stress is primarily a matter of learning to identify and modify the upsetting thoughts that are the cause of your upsetting feelings.

documented fact that personality and consciousness are made up of mental images, and that to correct psychological problems, you must identify and change these distorted images. Thus, guided imagery as a clinical tool involves your paying special attention to the specific images needed to bring about the changes in behavior that you desire. Imagery can be taught either individually or in groups, and a therapist will often use it to help bring about a specific result (for example, enhanced immune functioning during cancer, cessation of smoking, improved diet).

Practices that have a component of imagery are practically universal. These include systematic desensitization, REBT, biofeedback, hypnosis, neurolinguistic programming, gestalt therapy, and many others. In fact, any therapy that relies on imagination, visualization, or fantasy to communicate, motivate, solve problems, or increase awareness can be labeled a form of imagery. Moreover, types of meditation that include reciting a mantra or focusing attention on an imaginary object can also be considered a form of imagery, as can relaxation techniques and autogenic training that involve visualization (for example, "Your hands are heavy").

Imagery consists of two major processes: *evaluation* and *mental rehearsal*. Evaluation involves your being asked to describe your condition, as in "How do you feel?" This is usually done early in sessions, setting the stage for the rest of therapy. Mental rehearsal is then used to relieve anxiety and pain prior to an anxiety-provoking event. For example, surgery or a difficult treatment can be mentally rehearsed beforehand so that you're prepared and feel less anxious. Normally, a relaxation procedure is also taught, as are other coping techniques, like distraction and deep breathing. In many instances, mental rehearsal can lessen the pain, discomfort, and side effects associated with medical conditions and treatments.

Hypnosis

Hypnosis is an altered state of consciousness, a trancelike state, in which responsiveness to suggestions is heightened and the recall of hidden memories becomes easier. Recent opinion considers the phenomenon of a "hypnotic trance" to be a very relaxed mental state that can be attained through guided imagery and meditation.

Hypnotherapy relies on the use of suggestions to induce change. Persons wanting to be hypnotized visit a clinical *hypnotherapist* and undergo *hypnotic induction*, in which they're instructed to relax and "go inside" the mind. In other words, hypnosis involves an ability to set aside critical judgment without relinquishing it completely, as well as an ability to make believe and fantasize.

It's important to understand a couple of things about hypnosis. First, hypnosis isn't mind control or brainwashing. Second, the effectiveness of hypnotic suggestion has less to do with the skills of the hypnotist and more to do with the suggestibility and personality of the person hypnotized. Third, hypnosis can't cause you to act against your will or contradict your values. A hypnotherapist is ethically required to make only those suggestions that you've both decided are in your best interest. You won't be asked to do things that go against your morals or values. The idea that a hypnotized person is an automaton, is unable to resist any suggestion that is given, or won't be able to wake up from a trance is completely based on Hollywood-type misconceptions rather than factual information. While hypnotized persons are susceptible to suggestion, there are definite limits.

Hypnosis has many clinical applications and is well-documented as a therapy by psychological, psychiatric, medical, and dental associations around the globe. In the mental health field, hypnosis is widely used. For instance, revivifying traumatic events continues to be a useful treatment for relieving anxiety caused by traumas (for example, following combat, rape, natural disaster). In the medical field, hypnosis is quite helpful in preparing patients for anesthesia, reducing required drug dosages, alleviating a pregnant mother's discomfort during childbirth, and managing otherwise intractable pain (for example, from cancer). It's also used to treat high blood pressure, headaches, and many other conditions. And in dentistry, hypnosis is invaluable for reducing dental fears.

Given all of these benefits, hypnosis—especially when applied in combination with REBT—can be an exceptionally powerful tool for treating health anxiety syndrome.

Biofeedback

Biofeedback is based on the principle that our minds have an innate potential to control, at least to a certain degree, the autonomic functions of our bodies. For instance, in a matter of hours or days you can be trained to change the temperature of your hands, at will, by five to ten degrees. You can learn to alter your brain waves, reduce the frequency of asthma or allergy attacks, or manage pain. You can even be trained to prevent a migraine headache by diverting the blood that ordinarily engorges the blood vessels of your head to your hands and arms. Various controlled trials and a number of field studies have shown that biofeedback therapy can effectively induce relaxation and reduce some of the complications associated with irritable bowel syndrome, tension headaches, and stroke. In other words, you can be taught to control the allegedly involuntary processes (for example, blood pressure, heart rate) that increase when you're under stress.

Biofeedback relies on equipment with specialized sensors that track skin temperature, muscle contractions, and brain waves. The biofeedback machine "feeds back" your efforts at control in the form of a signal (such as a buzz). Once you're connected to the biofeedback machine, you're instructed to extinguish the signal (which is often annoying by design). Because you have no idea what to do, you must rely on trial and error to determine how to relax and, thus, stop the signal. In this way, you eventually learn to control your responses to stress without the equipment. Most biofeedback sessions are scheduled weekly and last from thirty to sixty minutes.

Several types of biofeedback machines provide information about the systems in your body that are affected by stress. These include *GSR, temperature feedback, EMG,* and *EEG* machines.

GSR. *Galvanic skin response* (GSR) training (also called *electrodermal response,* or *EDR*) measures the skin's electrical conductance, which is related to sweat gland activity. You probably know this form of biofeedback from its use in so-called lie detector tests. As a minute electrical current is applied to your skin, the GSR equipment measures changes in the levels of water and salt released from your sweat glands. The more emotionally aroused you are, the more active your sweat glands are, and the greater your skin's electrical conductivity is. GSR is frequently used for anxiety, phobias, stress, panic, excessive sweating, stuttering, and poor athletic performance.

Temperature feedback. *Temperature feedback* utilizes a machine that monitors skin temperature. A sensor is attached to a finger of your dominant hand or to a toe. If you're anxious or nervous, your skin temperature will drop as blood redirects from your hands and feet to your internal organs and muscles. Temperature feedback can be invaluable for treating stress, migraine headaches, and circulatory disorders like Raynaud's disease, which is characterized by excessively cold hands and feet.

EMG. An *electromyogram* (EMG) measures muscle tension. Two electrodes (or sensors) are taped onto your skin over the muscle to be monitored (for example, your jaw muscle). When the electrodes measure muscle tension, the device produces a buzz, beep, or colored light. You can hear or see continuous monitoring of your muscle's activity as you learn what tension feels like as it begins to mount. Then you can eliminate the tension before it worsens or causes physical problems. EMG seems particularly good for treating neck pain, jaw pain, tension headaches, backache, and stress-related conditions like ulcers and asthma.

EEG. An *electroencephalogram* (EEG) monitors brain wave activity. Because *alpha waves* are characteristic of states of relaxation (versus *beta waves*, which are characteristic of states of wakefulness), you might find relief from anxiety, stress, insomnia, and perhaps epilepsy by learning to increase your alpha wave activity. EEG seems to be more effective when used as an adjunct to other methods.

Biofeedback is likely to be more effective when combined with relaxation techniques and cognitive behavioral psychotherapy. That way, you can learn how to control your reactions to stress while also exploring how your thinking and behaviors contribute to it.

You can purchase biofeedback instruments for use at home. The most affordable ones are designed to monitor only one response, such as skin conductivity.

Homework Assignments

Your progress in therapy will depend largely on what you do outside of sessions. To assist you in making the most of any therapy experience, your therapist will probably assign you numerous *homework assignments*. At the start of each session, your therapist will review your progress as reflected in these assignments. It's normal not to want to do homework (just ask most teenagers!). However, if you keep refusing to do as the therapist suggests, you might want to decide if, somehow, you're engaging in *self-sabotaging behavior* and getting in the way of your own progress by not properly engaging in therapy. You might also want to consider what secondary gains you're receiving from not doing your homework. Always feel free to discuss any aspect of your homework assignments with your therapist.

Typical psychological homework assignments might include:

Reading assignments. Also referred to as *bibliotherapy*, reading is central to most therapeutic homework. Assignments might include reading books, articles, workbook materials, or information on the Internet. Reading, in and of itself, isn't probably sufficient to rid yourself of health anxiety syndrome. But it can be a great adjunct to other therapies, such as the CBT techniques described in this book.

Experiential assignments. It's not enough for most of us to simply think about our irrational cognitive distortions. To eliminate long-held beliefs, it's necessary to dispute them vigorously, which also means rationally acting and emoting in your everyday life. Here are a few common REBT methods for accomplishing this:

- *Risk taking:* This involves taking risks by directly confronting your fears to eliminate them.

- *Discomfort tolerance:* Here, you subject yourself to unpleasant, annoying situations to practice not upsetting yourself. A good example is intentionally driving into a huge, tangled traffic jam to learn frustration tolerance.

- *Attacking shame:* This involves countering embarrassment and shame by being silly—that is, doing something that would typically embarrass you but not hurt anyone else. Try making a spontaneous speech in the park, or break out into song while on the subway. These types of experiences will prove you don't need others' approval or respect.

- *Attacking perfectionism:* Here, you battle your perfectionistic tendencies by purposely doing things imperfectly. Some good examples are shaving only part of your face, not making your bed, leaving dirty dishes in the sink, and not washing your car after driving through mud.

Written assignments. Written homework also helps in your recovery from health anxiety syndrome. These assignments might take the form of keeping a journal, answering workbook questions, filling out your Cognitive Reframing Form, or all three. You'll probably find it's easiest to set aside about thirty minutes every day to write out your homework assignments, which you'll then bring to sessions for your therapist to review.

Many people express strong feelings—from boredom to apprehension to excitement—when it comes to doing therapeutic homework assignments. It's good to discuss these feelings openly with your therapist. Although homework assignments can be uncomfortable or downright frustrating, you'll find you receive much more from therapy if you take the time to do them.

For Personal Reflection

Which of the above homework assignments would you feel comfortable doing? Not feel comfortable doing? Why?

Therapy Formats

Finally, I want you to know that the therapies described in this chapter can be administered within various formats. The two most popular are *individual therapy* and *group therapy*, both of which differ from *self-help therapy* (described in the feature following this book's Introduction).

Individual Therapy

Individual therapy typically includes weekly one-on-one meetings with a psychologist, psychiatrist, counselor, social worker, or other mental health professional. This type of therapy provides you with a chance to process such important issues as anxiety, stress, depression, self-doubt, dissatisfaction, shyness, sexual and relationship problems, family conflicts, educational difficulties, drug and alcohol abuse, eating disorders, or virtually any other concern. Most of us have been troubled by something at one point or another in our lives. If you're experiencing significant discomfort that requires help beyond the suggestions provided in this book, you should consider seeking personal counseling. There's no reason to feel embarrassed. Going in for some individual therapy is perhaps the most responsible step you can take to rid yourself of health anxieties, as well as most any other psychological problem.

Group Therapy

Group therapy typically includes weekly meetings with one or two mental health professionals and a small number of clients. The idea is to work toward understanding and resolving various concerns within a group context. Whereas you might believe your problems can best be addressed in individual counseling, a therapy group's support, input, and feedback can be unparalleled in terms of helping all members develop awareness and overcome life hurdles. How? In group therapy, you have an opportunity to examine your reactions to a range of people, to experiment with new ways of interacting, and to practice giving and receiving appropriate feedback.

One special form of group therapy is *couple's therapy*, which is designed to deal with conflicts or relationship problems peculiar to spouses or partners. Generally speaking, a couple meets together with their therapist for weekly sessions. Many couples have had their relationship negatively impacted by health anxiety syndrome, and thus find it helpful to seek out relationship counseling.

For Personal Reflection

Which therapy format would you prefer for addressing your health anxieties?

Conclusions

In this chapter, I've introduced you to a wide range of techniques for conquering your fears of symptoms and disease. Each approach can be used alone or in combination, though most require the expertise of a licensed clinician. In my experiences with clients, I've consistently found that starting with self-help cognitive therapy methods is best, followed by adding behavioral and medical methods when the situation warrants it. In other words, try solving your problems on your own first, and then seek professional help if you decide you need more.

In the next chapter, we look at how people with health anxiety syndrome can benefit from the support of family and friends.

Feature: To Be or Not to Be . . . A Mental Disorder

The topic of self-help treatment of health anxiety syndrome frequently brings up the question of whether a problem, condition, or syndrome is a *mental disorder* as conceptualized by the American Psychiatric Association, which publishes the *Diagnostic and Statistical Manual of Mental Disorders*. For your information, then, I present a few of the basic principles involved in the process of diagnosing mental illnesses.

What Is Psychopathology?

Psychopathology (or *abnormal psychology*) is the scientific study of psychological disorders, which are specific patterns of ineffective thoughts and behaviors that cause distress and interfere with effective daily living. Abnormal psychology is a field within the overall discipline of psychology.

Determining Abnormality

Deciding what is abnormal versus normal behavior isn't always an easy task. Many experts have suggested that multiple factors can help determine whether behavior is abnormal or not. The most popular of these are maladaptiveness, harmfulness, statistical prevalence, personal distress, and sociocultural norms.

Maladaptiveness and harmfulness. *Maladaptiveness* is dysfunctional, and therefore fails to promote the psychological health, welfare, and fulfillment of the person. Maladaptive behavior can find many expressions, such as the inability to leave home (as in agoraphobia), drug addiction, and depression. *Harmfulness* usually refers to destructiveness, whether directed at the self or others. Being a threat disrupts a person's ability to function easily and reasonably in society.

Statistical rarity. Many types of mental disorders are *statistically rare* occurrences in that the vast majority of the people in a given society or culture don't experience them. For example, most Americans don't engage in compulsive hand-washing rituals as do people with obsessive-compulsive disorder. Nor do most Americans hear imaginary voices as do people with schizophrenia.

Personal distress. One criterion of psychopathology, *personal distress*, isn't always as noticeable or severe as you might expect. Some of us are adept at hiding our discomfort, whether it involves shame, guilt, grief, anxiety, anger, disappointment, or job stress. Plus, most people can relate to experiencing any or all of these at some point. The difference becomes one of the intensity of the distress.

Sociocultural norms. Societies and cultures create *norms* concerning which behaviors are acceptable and which aren't. And what is considered normal or abnormal can vary considerably across groups. In other words, what is normal for one society might be abnormal for another. Norm-violating behavior can signal that an individual is in psychological trouble.

Definitions of abnormality can also change across time, including from one historical period to another. For instance, masturbation is now seen as a normal expression of sexuality instead of a cause of insanity, as was commonly thought a mere 100 years ago in this country.

Classifying Mental Disorders

At the heart of clinical psychology is *diagnosis*, or the process whereby psychologists and psychiatrists classify abnormal behavior. Today's standard for this is the American Psychiatric Association's DSM, the first edition of which was published in 1952. The DSM's system of classification has undergone continuous refinement. The current DSM-IV-TR (2000) is based on available scientific research in its support of its various diagnostic categories.

Advantages and disadvantages of diagnosis. It's important to consider the many benefits of classifying mental disorders. First, a diagnostic system offers clinicians agreed-upon standards for understanding and using diagnostic labels to describe abnormal behavior. Second, a classification system assists psychologists in making predictions about disorders, including who is vulnerable, as well as their *prognosis* (chances of recovery). Third, a diagnostic system offers psychologists the opportunity to devise theories about the causes of and treatments for specific disorders.

But not all psychologists advocate using diagnostic labels like the ones in the DSM-IV-TR. Critics claim, for example, that labeling people as "mentally ill" encourages them to perceive themselves and act as if they're "mentally ill." It also invites them to assume a "sick role" as an excuse for avoiding regular responsibilities and not facing up to their problems.

Even though the details of mental health diagnosis and treatment are confidential, many individuals fear repercussions should their diagnoses become known to others. This is even more the case when clinicians rely on insurance and other third-party payers that process claims by inputting treatment information into computer databases. If patients fear others will gain access to such databases, they may forego seeking badly needed mental health therapy.

Using a diagnostic system with members of racial minority groups can also be problematic, especially when the therapists' and clients' differing cultural backgrounds affect the outcome of mental health assessment and diagnosis. For example, a Caucasian psychologist might not recognize that minimal eye contact among some Asian clients is a sign of respect, and not a symptom of depression or social anxiety.

Finally, continuing revisions of the DSM have reflected advancements in scientific knowledge about the classification of mental disorders. On the basis of research and clinical experience, the authors of the DSM have added, dropped, or revised diagnostic categories with each successive edition, which has on occasion generated controversy among clinicians and researchers alike. One example was the controversy that initially surrounded the APA's 1973 decision to remove homosexuality as a mental disorder from the DSM's classification system. Another example was the controversy over the APA's decision to eliminate the term neurosis, which has traditionally referred to relatively mild mental disorders in which an individual is able to maintain contact with reality.

Question for Thought: Given what you've just read about some of the intricacies of mental health diagnosis, when might—or might not—health anxieties be considered a mental disorder?

6

The Role of Family, Friends, and Support Groups

People must help one another; it is nature's law.

—Jean de la Fontaine

John Donne perhaps said it best when he wrote, "No man is an island." Indeed, as social beings we live around other people, and we need other people.

Remember the *systems perspective* that I described in chapter 2? This view of life is concerned with the *interacting systems* in which most of us live. In this chapter, we focus on the role that family members, friends, coworkers, colleagues, acquaintances, and significant others can play in your recovery from health anxiety syndrome. I'll also speak to what significant others can do for themselves and their loved ones, as well as offer a few comments concerning the benefits of educational classes and support groups (such as twelve-step groups like Emotions Anonymous).

In previous chapters, I've commented that you're in charge of your own life and circumstances. However, I'm not suggesting that looking to others for help is a cop-out. Yes, you're ultimately responsible for your own thoughts, emotions, and behaviors. But a large part of taking responsibility for your own recovery is acknowledging those important interconnections with your fellow human beings, and drawing support from your interpersonal relationships.

"In Our Secrets Lie Our Sicknesses"

This particular quote is well-known among those who've participated in various forms of group work. Many years ago, I worked at an inpatient treatment center for addictions where I learned an important principle of recovery from psychological problems: *You can't do it totally on your own.* In this particular setting, the patients learned this principle by participating in many daily counseling and support groups. Day by day, we all saw that without sharing our problems and asking for help, we can't get "unstuck" from our dysfunctional patterns.

Even if you do nothing more than read a book like this one, you're still looking outside of yourself for some ideas. And that's the way it should be. If you don't look outside yourself, your inner "light bulb" probably won't light up. And even if you do find some insights within the recesses of your psyche, that doesn't mean you're opening yourself up to the fullest opportunities for self-improvement.

Should You Ask for Support?

Yes! The simple reality is that, without any intervention, health anxiety can—and does—ruin lives and relationships. And as I've shown throughout this book, if you have health anxiety, you've probably been resistant to seeking help. This is where having a support network of family and friends can prove to be of immense value. Of course, support people have their own emotional needs, challenges, and confusions. I'll speak to this issue shortly.

For those who've never experienced health anxiety syndrome, the problem might not seem like such a big deal. So what if a loved one worries all the time about her health? So what if a boyfriend compulsively exercises for hours every day to avoid having a heart attack? So what if a spouse can't sleep? So what if a parent makes frequent visits to doctors? After all, it's not like health anxiety is a real problem, right? Think again! Living with the constant fear that serious disease is present, that no one is listening, and that death is imminent can be a highly disconcerting problem.

Unfortunately, being fearful of diseases or germs can become a virtual full-time distraction—a preoccupation. If you miss work often because of sicknesses or frequent medical appointments, the syndrome can affect your job. If you turn down social invitations because you're always sick or don't want to catch germs from other people, it can affect your social life. If you "burn out" family members and friends by repeatedly relying on them to take you to the doctor or pick up prescriptions, it can affect your relationships. If you jog obsessively and hurt your knees, it can affect your health. If you spend a lot of money on medications, co-payments, or excessive lab tests, it can affect your finances. In short, health anxiety literally can intrude into all aspects of life. Nor is there a place to hide from your health worries. They're with you around the clock.

Because health anxieties are so often met with disbelief or criticism, you're probably hesitant to ask significant others for help. The people around you certainly know you've got a problem. Nonetheless, openly admitting to fear and asking for support and cooperation can be tough, because you're never quite sure how others will react. *But you can do it!* Remember, even though you don't need anyone else's approval, you can benefit from their help.

This means . . . *ask, ask, ask!* You're not alone, and those who truly care for you will be there to help regardless of your problems.

Now let's take a quick look at some of the ways family members can support you. I've addressed the rest of this chapter directly to your loved ones, so you can pass the book along to them or make photocopies of these pages.

Practical Pointer

Perhaps the most critical factor in determining a disease phobic's ability to ask for help from loved ones is effective communication, which involves quality talking and listening. Beyond the mere transmission of information, communication helps people better understand and relate to each other. It helps them feel warm, close, and connected. It creates an atmosphere of mutual cooperation in which active problem-solving can take place.

Effective communication can also do much to reduce the common relationship tensions that arise in response to health anxiety syndrome. People usually find it easier to work through relationship problems when they're able to communicate honestly as a couple. This includes dealing with the exhaustion and frustration that loved ones so often feel when a significant other has health anxieties.

What Can You Do If You Know Someone with Health Anxiety?

How can you as a family member, friend, coworker, or significant other best assist someone with health anxiety? The first thing you can do is not be critical or judgmental about health anxiety. Don't minimize the condition or belittle the person. Instead, thoughtfully and attentively listen to what the disease phobic has to say about his or her fears, experiences, and goals for recovery. Express compassion without showing pity or being patronizing.

Negative comments or criticism from family members often make health anxieties worse, whereas calm, supportive comments can help improve outcomes. If your loved one views your help as interference, remember that it's probably the health anxiety talking. Try to be as patient and kind as possible. Demanding that a loved one with health anxiety syndrome just stop worrying about their health usually doesn't help; it can also make her or him feel worse because this kind of compliance isn't possible. Rather, applaud all successful attempts to resist giving into health worries. That is, build on positives rather than tear down negatives!

Don't push too hard. You shouldn't expect too much improvement too soon. The problem didn't appear overnight, and it's not going to disappear overnight either. Keep in mind that no one dislikes health anxieties more than the person who has this problem.

After gains have been made, be cognizant of any telltale signs of relapse. If health anxieties are beginning to reappear, you'll probably become aware of it first. Be sure to point out early symptoms in a thoughtful manner.

Never forget that your reactions can have an enormous impact—positive or negative—on whether or not the other person will admit there's nothing physically wrong and then try to solve his or her problems. If you respond with derision or mimicry, the disease phobic will either 1) abandon beneficial behaviors that lead to recovery, or 2) complain of an exacerbation of physical symptoms and anxieties! In contrast, if you respond with sensitivity and empathy, his or her fears of being criticized or judged will diffuse, setting the stage for healthy changes and improvement to begin. The subject of health anxiety is a sensitive topic, so being a considerate listener and active helper will do much to provide the support that is so necessary for recovery.

Following are ten additional suggestions on how you can be a useful resource to someone with health anxiety syndrome:

1. Support the person by not enabling them. In particular, don't promote doctor shopping, scheduling unnecessary medical appointments and tests, using unnecessary medications, exercising excessively, or exerting extreme dietary controls.

2. Support the disease phobic by taking an active role in his or her self-help treatment. Try offering encouragement, helping with completion of the Cognitive Reframing Chart, or providing an environment that encourages long-term healing.

3. Acknowledge and praise the phobic's accomplishments—whether large or small—based on individual goals rather than absolute standards.

4. Keep stress levels (at home, work, etc.) to a minimum.

5. When children or teenagers have health anxieties, be sure to work with school nurses, teachers, and administrators to make sure they understand the syndrome. As is the case with any child with a problem, parents must set uniform limits so the child or adolescent knows what is expected of them.

6. Accept the fact that in-person counseling might be warranted. If this is the case, be willing to take an active role in the therapeutic process. Many mental health professionals recommend the inclusion of significant others in treatment, especially in more severe situations. The exact nature of your assistance will vary according to the actual problems and your relationship with the patient. You might, for example, accompany the patient into anxiety-producing situations during graduated exposure sessions. Also, health anxiety behaviors (for example, multiple late-night visits to the ER) tend to stress out family members, which is another reason why it's often necessary for them to participate in therapy with the patient.

7. Be open to exploring family and/or marital issues that have arisen in response to your loved one's health anxieties.

8. Assist him or her in completing homework that the therapist has assigned. This could include, for example, helping her or him practice shame-attacking exercises or anti-perfectionism activities.

9. Keep in mind that the recovery process is frequently a source of tension, primarily because it changes existing relationships. People's emotional needs and reactions frequently change during the course of treatment. Living through these changes requires patience while everyone works toward more stable and satisfying relationships.

10. Read whatever educational materials are available so that you stay as informed as possible.

For Personal Reflection

Which of the suggestions given above do you think might prove most helpful for you, given your unique situation?

The Impact of Health Anxiety on Significant Others

Without a doubt, it's the individual with health anxiety syndrome who suffers the most intensely. Yet, we often forget the other victims of this problem: the caretakers, family members, and friends whose lives are also negatively affected by this perplexing syndrome. As such, significant others may have a hard time finding a place to express their concerns or process their strong feelings about living with someone who has excessive health worries. As one man described it:

> For many years, my health anxieties have stressed my marriage. It's difficult for anyone, even a spouse, who's never experienced the terror of worrying about deadly diseases to understand. I've never been able to completely explain it to my wife. On the one hand, it all sounds so irrational. I mean, in my heart, I know I'm not dying from cancer, AIDS, or some mysterious virus. On the other hand, though, I just can't seem to stop thinking about my symptoms, even though most everything else in my life is fine. I know my wife has a hard time. She's tried over and over, without much success, to reassure me. On good days, she makes sense. But most of the time I just can't let go to believe it. It can't be that simple. I know she gets very annoyed with me. We're both reading about health anxieties, and also talking a lot more. My wife is also going to a support group, so now she has a place to vent her frustrations."

Indeed, resentment and hurt feelings can build over the years and strain marriages and other relationships. A disease phobic's behavior can even create serious hurt feelings and misunderstandings. According to the husband of one patient:

> My wife has worn me out with her worries about having a disease. I've tried endlessly to convince her that she's okay. Otherwise, the 10 zillion exams and tests she's undergone would've shown something! I'd say my main hassle is that I feel negated, like my opinion doesn't count with her. She doesn't listen to me or her doctors. I'm also tired of spending all our spare time—time we could be doing something fun—driving to hospitals or sitting in doctors' offices.

And as one woman noted:

> It gets difficult when I have to work and take care of everything at home—kids, schools, activities, and meals—when my husband is having one of his "attacks."

There can also be problems in the bedroom:

> Mary has virtually killed our sex life. My every advance
> for sex is met with comments like, "I feel sick," "I hurt,"
> or "I'm too exhausted." Who gets in the mood that way?
> These days, I'm lucky if she's willing to make love once
> or twice every six months. It's very frustrating!

Although it's important that disease phobics receive understanding, caring, and love, it's just as important that significant others receive the same.

Sometimes, the person with health anxieties continues to refuse to face the problem. If your loved one doesn't want to address their worry, there is little that you can do to force them:

> My brother just won't come around. He simply can't
> handle the idea that he's not dying from some weird
> microorganism. He evidently thinks that he'd be seen as
> less of a man if he has a mental problem than if he has
> a "real disease." I totally disagree, but we did grow up in
> a very macho household where men must never show any
> weakness. You pull yourself up by your own bootstraps.
> And there was no such thing as mental illness in our
> parents' world. At this point, my brother seems content
> to continue living with his fears rather than facing them.
> I've offered to help him, but he won't listen. I guess there's
> nothing much I can do.

Many family members and significant others are confused and frustrated by the symptoms of health anxiety syndrome. They don't know how to help their loved one, and they don't know where to get support for themselves. As one man complained:

> What can you possibly do when your wife gets a nosebleed
> in the middle of the night, and then decides to rush to the
> emergency room thinking her brain is hemorrhaging?

Taking Care of Yourself

If you live with a disease phobic, you know how exhausting the situation can become. So, be certain to make time for yourself. It's necessary to continue to lead your own life and avoid becoming a prisoner of your loved one's fears and behaviors. If you're not totally burned out, you'll be in a much better position to provide the support needed to help in your loved one's recovery.

Here are ten suggestions on how to take care of yourself when a loved one has health anxiety syndrome:

1. Do everything possible to help your significant other overcome his or her own problems, but freely accept your limitations. Bear in mind that we can only change ourselves; we can't change other people.

2. Don't allow the disease phobic's problems to take center stage all of the time. You have needs, too.

3. Keep alert to signs of depression. If you feel depressed, talk to someone who can help you—a friend, a pastor, or a counselor.

4. Trust your instincts. Know when to stop the insanity of doctor shopping, useless medical tests, exercise addictions, and so on. Also, know when to speak up and say, "There's a problem here!"

5. Learn as much as you can about your loved one's syndrome.

6. Keep an open mind about new ways to promote the disease phobic's recovery.

7. Look for support from other people who are in similar situations. Knowing that you're not alone can be quite empowering.

8. Attend a group like Emotions Anonymous. Take advantage of whatever help is available. Sharing your thoughts and experiences with others who have gone through the same things can be a big help. Support groups are a good way to learn new strategies for coping and assisting loved ones and to feel less alone. (See the Resources section at the end of this book for some addresses and phone numbers.)

9. Love, respect, and value yourself as an individual.

10. Above all else, take care of yourself. Living with a health phobic can be challenging. This means you deserve some quality time alone.

Conclusions

As a person with health anxieties, you need to accept the fact there's no shame in seeking help from your family and friends. Yes, you're in charge of exercising intentional conscious control to improve yourself. You're in charge of changing your own thoughts, feelings, and

Practical Pointer

A support group is a gathering of people who regularly meet to discuss and process common life issues or problems. A group might include a health-care provider as facilitator, or it might be led by its members. Most support groups are formed to help those who suffer from a particular condition or disease. Perhaps the best-known example of a support group is Alcoholics Anonymous, whose twelve-step program has helped countless alcoholics attain sobriety and remain abstinence.

behaviors. You're in charge of recognizing your own personal flaws and deciding to master your circumstances and your life. But you can also speed up the process of your recovery by enlisting the aid of those around you. This isn't a sign of weakness; it's a sign of your motivation to heal, as well as your commitment to eradicate health anxieties from your life.

As a significant other, you can help the person with health anxiety syndrome by accepting what's really going on. A disease phobic's denial of a problem and/or refusal to change can become quite a challenge. In some cases, you might want to schedule a family meeting to discuss your impressions of the situation, much as is done with alcoholic family members who are in denial.

You can play a vital role in your loved one's recovery. Demonstrating sensitivity and comprehension of the immense impact that health anxieties can have, remaining uncritical and nonjudgmental of the syndrome, being an attentive listener, and taking care of yourself are all effective ways to support your loved one's struggle against health anxiety syndrome.

Feature: Handling Criticism

If you have health anxiety, you might be hesitant to tell family and friends about your problem for fear of criticism and rejection. After all, if you've had a physician accuse you of "faking" your symptoms or an acquaintance derogatorily call you a "hypochondriac," you're probably unwilling to risk sharing your personal problems with *anyone* to avoid being unfairly criticized.

No one truly enjoys criticism, especially when it seems that the other person's intent is to hurt or manipulate. But like so many of the potential negatives I've described in *Stop Worrying About Your Health!*, it's not the intent or nature of the criticism that makes the difference; it's how you interpret and accept it. In other words, you can look at criticism as a threat to your self-esteem, or you can consider the source, forget about it, and go on about your business. It might be *unpleasant* when a relative accuses you of spending too much time at the doctor's office, but it's not *awful*. You don't *have* to believe what she says. She might think you're faking illnesses to get attention, but there's no golden rule that requires you to see things the same way she does.

I mentioned at the start of this chapter that I believe in the saying, "In our secrets lie our sicknesses." By this I mean it's beneficial for you to seek support from those around you, even if it means you might be faced with uncomfortable remarks. During my years in practice, I've noticed a tendency for people with health anxiety syndrome to be unusually sensitive to other people's criticism. I know it's hard to trust others, especially if you've had bad experiences in the past.

The ability to handle criticism without "losing it" is a useful skill to add to your repertoire of psychological strategies. But before going any further, I think it's helpful to distinguish between two types of criticism: *constructive* (friendly) and *destructive* (unfriendly). The first is meant to be helpful, is normally delivered by someone who cares about you and your feelings, and is generally welcome. The second is hurtful, delivered by someone who doesn't care, and is never welcome. Constructive criticism can be quite valuable. Its main intent is to help you learn a thing or two about yourself, develop as an individual, or enhance your performance in a particular area.

Destructive criticism is neither valuable nor helpful. Its main intent is to malign, belittle, and control you. When people think about the concept of criticism, they tend to conjure up the negative images and feelings associated with the destructive type.

Dealing effectively with either type of criticism involves knowing what to think, say, and do. One of the first questions you want to ask yourself when criticized is, "Is this person's criticism valid?" Many times people give each other constructive criticism because they care about and want to help each other. There's always the possibility that a particular criticism *could be true*. Then again, people are imperfect and sometimes offer one another erroneous criticism. Only you can decide what you'll accept as true and what you won't. In the end, regardless of the content of the criticism, it's always important to remember that we're all entitled to our own opinions.

Let's take a closer look at how this works. If Christie tells George she thinks he's afraid to attend a local support group for phobics, George would ask himself, "Am I afraid of attending a support group for phobics?" If he answers "Yes," he doesn't need to start a fight with Christie, or berate himself for being a fallible human being. George can choose to accept his wife's comments as constructive feedback and an opportunity for personal growth. If, however, George's answer is "No" to the question, he still doesn't need to get angry or down on himself or Christie. George keeps in mind that Christie, like himself, is a fallible human being, and is subject to making the same sorts of mistakes as he makes. Neither Christie nor George might ever be able to prove who is right on the particular topic of support groups, but they can agree it's okay to have differing opinions.

At the heart of many disease phobics' oversensitivity to criticism lie numerous *musts* of perfection, approval, and comfort. Learning to tolerate criticism, then, involves rigorously disputing and challenging your cognitive distortions of *demandingness*. Three very typical irrational beliefs related to oversensitivity to criticism are:

1. I *must* be absolutely perfect in every respect; otherwise I'm a bad person, and no one will love me.

2. Others *must* accept and approve of me in every respect; otherwise, I'm not a good person, and life isn't worth living.

3. I *must* only hear what I want to hear, because I can't tolerate the discomfort of listening to someone tell me about my faults.

It's also helpful not to take criticism personally, which is what most of us tend to do. Typically, the person making criticisms is actually making remarks about something you're *doing*, not about who you are as an individual. The trouble begins when you *personalize* criticism—when you apply what the other person says about your behavior to your self-worth. If you're ever tempted to do this, just remember that *you aren't what other people say or think*. Just because someone claims you're a "crock" doesn't mean *you actually are*. Why believe you're a villainous or bad person just because someone else says so? Stick to the facts, and ignore the rest of it. You'll save yourself a lot of headaches (pun intended!).

Questions for Thought: As someone with health anxiety, are you overly sensitive to the criticisms of others? Why might this be?

7

Future Directions

Natural forces within us are the true healers of disease.

—Hippocrates

My work in clinical mind-body psychology eventually piqued my interest in an entirely different area of health care that's collectively known by such phrases as *holistic health*, *integrative health*, *new age health*, *complementary medicine*, *alternative medicine*, *integral medicine*, and *blended medicine*. (I prefer the descriptors *complementary* and *integrative*, which imply that these methods have a place alongside of mainstream medical ones.) I've been particularly intrigued by the fact that *most complementary therapies promote attaining general wellness over correcting disease states*. Although these and other terms and ideas might cause some of my conventional readers to cringe, the fact remains that many forms of health care have existed throughout the world—most of them flourishing long before the development of what is referred to in the West as *allopathic medicine*.

Just because a therapy or technique has been around for a long time doesn't make it legitimate. But its longevity doesn't make it obsolete either. It's possible, for example, that the accumulated knowledge of the last 3,000 years of Oriental medicine has important insights to offer the West with regard to herbal formulas. (Don't forget that many of our standard pharmaceuticals, like their herbal counterparts, are based on plant derivatives.) I believe today's health-care system has much to learn from the practices of the past and from around the globe; we need to build on the best methods from both West and East. And to do this requires cooperation and mutual respect across disciplines and practitioners of differing backgrounds, as well as solidly designed, double-blind, controlled research studies. It won't happen overnight, but we can take some comfort in such developments as the National Institutes of Health having created an Office of Alternative Medicine to research the efficacy of various complementary methods.

Although I have enjoyed considerable training beyond my clinical psychology doctorate, I don't presume to be an expert in any of the complementary therapies. Nor do I believe a thorough review of three or four millennia's worth of medical history is within the scope of this book. A growing number of lay-oriented books are commercially available that describe nearly every aspect of Western and Eastern models of health care, including mainstream, complementary, psychological, and spiritual perspectives. Instead, this chapter is designed to serve as a very brief introduction to three models that might hold promise for sufferers of health anxiety syndrome. I've found these to be supported by Western scientific research methods. I also hope that this final chapter of *Stop Worrying About Your Health!* will show you the value of an *integral model* for overall health care—one that harmonizes care of the body, the mind, and the spirit.

Setting aside all of the political tangles associated with this topic, let's now consider how three prominent models of complementary health care—*massage therapy, chiropractic therapy,* and *Oriental medicine*—could be beneficial adjunctive therapies to the cognitive reframing techniques that I've already described.

Massage Therapy

As I've explained throughout *Stop Worrying About Your Health!*, stress causes bodily or mental tension that can become a factor in causing diseases, creating physical symptoms, and bringing on health anxieties. Your goal, then, should be to *manage* the stresses in your life, as it's impossible to completely eliminate stress. If you can learn to manage your stress and its effects, you can regain control over both your physical and mental health.

The last two decades have witnessed a tremendous surge of interest in *therapeutic massage therapy,* or the systematic manipulation of bodily soft tissues—in particular, the muscles—for the purpose of relaxing and "normalizing" their functioning to achieve optimum stress-reduction and wellness. In other words, a primary goal of massage therapy is to assist the body's ability to heal itself and to increase wellness by decreasing stress, bodily tension, and pain. Massage therapy has been incorporated into many health-care models, including both complementary and allopathic systems. Most massage therapists practice out of their own office, at spas and salons, at shopping malls, or in conjunction with other health-care practitioners, such as chiropractic doctors.

Massage therapy takes many forms, but three of the most common are *Swedish massage, deep tissue massage,* and *Tuina* (Chinese pressure point massage). Whatever the style practiced, massage therapists generally apply numerous massage strokes to eliminate muscle tension, including long and broad strokes, movable or fixed pressure, holding, percussion, and vibration. Whereas massage therapists mostly use their hands, some also use their forearms, elbows, feet, or mechanical devices to locate areas of tension and other soft-tissue problems, as well as manipulate soft tissues with the right amount of pressure (based on the client's feedback).

In massage therapy, *human touch* is central to the healing process. Touch conveys a sense of caring, compassion, and empathetic relationship—important ingredients in any form of mind-body healing. According to Frances Tappan (1988), author of *Healing Massage Techniques: Holistic, Classic, and Emerging Methods*:

> The art of healing is a two-way street. A massage given by one who includes the patient as partner will be remarkably more effective than that given as a mere technique of body manipulation. One who devotes total attention by communicating concern, empathy, and a sincere desire to promote the healing process will spur a patient to participate in the effort toward regaining health. (p. 35)

Interestingly, recent research in the form of several major papers has evaluated the effectiveness of massage for treating pain and found positive effects. For instance, one of the most convincing reports on the usefulness of massage appeared in an April 2001 issue of the *Archives of Internal Medicine* (Cherkin, Eisenberg, Sherman, et al. 2001).

Clinical Applications of Massage Therapy

What does massage therapy accomplish? From a physiological point of view, lactic acid can accumulate in overworked muscles, causing stiffness, pain, and even muscle spasm. Massage can assist in the elimination of this and other metabolic waste products. It improves circulation, which increases blood flow and delivers oxygen to bodily tissues, and it probably boosts immune functioning. Blocked, deadened areas are often able to respond to sensory input again. Massage also stimulates the release of *endorphins*—the body's own natural painkillers. All of these effects can speed healing after injury, enhance recovery from disease, and even prevent illnesses from developing in the first place.

From a psychological point of view, massage reduces stress and anxiety by promoting relaxation. During a massage, your tight muscles relax, and the pain associated with chronic tension is relieved. Massage also enhances self-esteem and promotes a general sense of well-being. As one friend remarked:

> *I've never bought into the holistic health thing, but after seeing some news reports on it, massage therapy seemed to make decent sense to me. I get pretty stressed out in my work as a textbook sales representative, so I decided to give massage a try. Well, it only took one professional massage for me to decide, this is it! Now I'm addicted.*

I get massages as often as I can afford them; they make me feel great!

Massage can reverse the damaging physiological effects of stress by helping to:

- Relax tense muscles

- Improve your circulation

- Lower your heart rate and blood pressure

- Heighten your personal sense of well-being

- Reduce your anxiety levels

As I described in chapter 5, a very powerful antidote to stress and anxiety is relaxation. During relaxation, your nervous and endocrine systems initiate bodily changes that slow your heart rate, lower your blood pressure, improve your circulation and digestion, and relax your muscles—all in counteraction to stress. A great many activities can bring about a relaxation response, including deep breathing, meditation, exercise, visualization, or listening to calming music. But, without a doubt, one of the best methods to battle stress and anxiety is therapeutic massage.

Massage and Health Anxiety Syndrome

Massage won't cure your health worries, but it might provide some welcome relief from the symptoms of anxiety, stress, and tension. Having regular massages will also put you in touch with your body, so that you're better able to monitor your body's signals of stress. Then you'll have a clearer idea of when your body is telling you it's time to rethink whatever is worrying you. Thus, massage can play a role in your recovery from health anxiety syndrome. By combining massage therapy with the cognitive techniques described in chapters 3 and 4, you can learn to avoid the damaging effects of chronic stress while also taking control of your psychological health.

Chiropractic Therapy

Chiropractic is a fast-growing branch of health care devoted to the idea that wellness depends, at least in part, on a normally functioning and healthy nervous system. Taken from the Greek words *cheir*

Practical Pointer

Having regular therapeutic massages can help you gain a clearer understanding of when your body is telling you it's time to rethink whatever is worrying you.

(meaning "hand") and *praxis* (meaning "practice"), *chiropractic* literally means "treatment by hand."

Doctors of chiropractic believe in the body's inherent wisdom to heal itself, and thus contend that the cause of many dysfunctional processes begins with the body's inability to adapt to its surroundings. Chiropractors look to address dysfunction, pain, and disease not by using medications or surgery, but by locating and correcting musculoskeletal areas of the body that are malfunctioning. This approach normally includes the fine art of *spinal adjustments*, in combination with massage therapy, nutritional modifications, lifestyle recommendations, exercise, and a wide range of other natural methods that promote physical and emotional fitness.

Why spinal adjustments? The human spinal column consists of a series of vertebrae (movable bones) extending from the base of the skull to the pelvis. Thirty-one pairs of spinal nerves continue from the brain down the spine, and these nerves exit through a series of openings in and between the vertebrae. As the nerves exit the spine, they form a complicated network that affects tissues in your body. Many everyday events can cause these spinal bones to lose their normal positioning. When this happens, a chain of events occurs that influences the spinal cord, nerves, muscles, and soft tissues. When the vertebrae remain out of alignment, the result is an impingement of the nerves that send messages throughout your body. Even small amounts of pressure on nerve roots can reduce the amount of neural transmission by as much as 50 percent.

What do spinal adjustments involve? According to Leon Coehlo's (1997) *Applied Chiropractic*:

> Traditional chiropractic . . . is characterized by specificity.
> The specific chiropractic adjustment is delivered via a short-lever, low force, high velocity thrust, applied to a specific vertebra or pelvic structure. The adjustment is actually the introduction of a force which the body then utilizes to place the vertebra in a normal biomechanical relationship with its neighbors. (p. 86)

In other words, the spinal vertebrae are realigned during a chiropractic adjustment. The desired result is a release of the impingement of the nerves, which then improves neural functioning.

Although chiropractic works for millions of people, the verdict is still out on exactly how it works. Many chiropractors speak of correcting the *vertebral subluxation complex* (misaligned vertebrae), while others speak of opening energy channels. Still others speak of restoring the motion of the vertebrae as they move against each other, as very subtle changes in the movement of vertebrae can have a significant effect on the nerves running through them. More research is needed to determine conclusively what underlies the effectiveness of spinal adjustments.

Clinical Applications of Chiropractic

The conditions that chiropractors address are as diverse as the human nervous system itself. For this reason, chiropractors rely on the same basic methods of physical examination, radiographic (X-ray) examination, laboratory analysis, consultation, and case history taking as any other physician. In addition, they use a standardized, comprehensive chiropractic structural examination while paying close attention to the alignment of the spinal vertebrae to determine a patient's condition and the appropriate course of therapy. This examination to evaluate the structural integrity and function of the spine is the hallmark of chiropractic, making it unique among the various health-care professions.

Chiropractic and Health Anxiety Syndrome

Living in our rigid and high-strung world causes many of us to develop muscular tensions that affect the psyche. This probably explains why so many patients who visit doctors of chiropractic describe stress and anxiety associated with their pain.

For reasons not exactly understood, stress and anxiety frequently strike the weaker areas of the spine, causing pain in the form of headaches, migraines, neck pain, back pain, and general muscular tension. This pain, in turn, ends up aggravating the stress, which then causes more pain. Why? When you have pain, your body and mind are under tremendous stress. You begin fretting, for example, about whether the pain will destroy your ability to work, sleep, have sex, and otherwise enjoy life. The stress increases nervous system activity, which in turns makes your subjective experience of pain feel more intense.

It stands to reason that stress and anxiety are also triggered by fears of anticipated pain (physical or emotional) and disability. Chiropractors and psychologists witness this phenomenon daily. That is, health anxiety can also result from the anticipation of physical problems, pain, and more anxiety. Chiropractic therapy is aimed at alleviating the musculoskeletal conditions that lead to, and aggravate, both physical *and* mental problems. In fact, patients frequently report reduced levels of anxiety and stress following chiropractic adjustments.

The manipulative process of chiropractic also allows some people to open up. When your tension is relieved, psychological issues and memories may surface. You then become more communicative about whatever it is that's bothering you.

Practical Pointer

Health anxiety can result from the anticipation of physical problems, pain, and more anxiety. Chiropractic therapy is aimed at alleviating the musculoskeletal conditions that lead to, and aggravate, both physical and mental problems.

Acupuncture and Oriental Medicine

An entirely distinct model of health care is *Oriental medicine*, a coordinated and complete system that is used to diagnose and treat sickness, prevent disease, and promote wellness. Also known as *traditional Chinese medicine* (TCM), Oriental medicine encompasses many diverse Asian health-enhancing and energy-balancing therapies. *Acupuncture* (from the Latin words *acus*, meaning "needle," and *punctura*, meaning "puncture") and *Chinese herbology* are probably the best-known techniques of Oriental medicine, and they're the ones I'll focus on here. Other frequently used TCM techniques include *Qigong, Guasha, Cupping, Moxibustion,* and *Tuina*— all of which involve ways to manipulate *Qi*—the essential energy of

life. Originating in China thousands of years ago, TCM is still practiced throughout the world today.

To comprehend the inner workings of TCM, it's helpful to
understand some of the basics of Chinese philosophy—a thorough
description of which is impractical for this book. The concepts of the
Tao, Yin and Yang, the Five Elements, and the Eight Principles are
all essential to TCM and its unique role in helping to maintain good
health, but can come across as rather intimidating to the first-time
reader. Fortunately, you don't need to understand Oriental medical
theory to benefit from Oriental medicine.

For the purposes of this discussion, one theory does bear men-
tioning. The view that we're each governed by the opposing but
complementary forces of Yin and Yang is at the core of Chinese philosophy. This balance of forces is thought to permeate and affect the
entire universe, including us. Thus, a primary goal of Oriental medicine is to restore the balance between your Yin and Yang in order to
restore health and to prevent illness. Their thorough understanding
of such concepts as Yin and Yang (and many others) allows TCM
practitioners to diagnose and treat a variety of conditions effectively.

Oriental medicine, then, looks at sickness as a state of being
"out of balance." That's why in TCM you're encouraged to examine
lifestyle, thinking, feelings, habits, and values in order to understand
your problem from a larger perspective. Your symptoms (whether
physical, mental, or both) are considered to be consequences of ineffective lifestyle habits, as well as your body's striving to restore
balance.

Eastern medicine differs considerably from Western medicine,
which often pursues symptom removal at all costs. Although the
elimination of symptoms is an important objective in TCM treatment,
it's not the ultimate one. Oriental medicine's aim is to restore function and balance. And because it's the patient's responsibility to pre-
serve his or her own wellness, patient education is an integral part of
Oriental medicine.

Practical Pointer

*Oriental medicine looks at sickness as a state of being
"out of balance." Thus, a primary goal of Oriental
medicine is to bring back the balance between your
Yin and Yang in order to restore health and to prevent
illness.*

And the Point? Acupuncture

Even though it's only one of numerous TCM techniques, acupuncture usually comes to mind when people talk about Oriental medicine. In and of itself, acupuncture is quite effective for treating physical and psychological problems.

The procedure originated in China more than 2,500 years ago and has continued to be refined since that time. Although Western health-care professionals often express skepticism at acupuncture, its proven potency has been recognized for millennia. On the topic of such skepticism, Felix Mann (1973) noted in his classic text, *Acupuncture: The Ancient Chinese Art of Healing and How It Works Scientifically*:

> The notion that a pinprick, often in a part of the body far removed from the seat of disease, can cure an illness is alien to conventional thinking. It is unfortunately the case that many doctors, even when faced with one or several patients who have been cured by acupuncture where there own efforts have been fruitless, refuse to believe the evidence . . . [However] much of what is factually observed in acupuncture could be explained in a way completely different from that of the traditional Chinese account. One example might be a different account by way of the discipline of neurophysiology. (pp. 1, 3)

Acupuncture involves the insertion of fine, sterilized needles about the size of a human hair into the skin to bring about therapeutic actions. Again, Oriental medicine views health as intimately related to Qi. When imbalances in the normal flow of Qi within the body occur, disease results. Along with the usual method of puncturing the skin with needles, practitioners also use heat, friction, pressure, suction, or impulses of electromagnetic energy to stimulate various *acupuncture points*, which are specific areas on the body that respond to needle stimulation.

The goal of acupuncture is to rebuild health by normalizing the flow of Qi through either *tonifying* or *sedating* specific acupuncture points. From a Western perspective, this could be explained as varying the electromagnetic fields of the human body. (Acupuncture points have been demonstrated to possess specific electrical properties, so that stimulating these points alters the levels of chemical neurotransmitters in the body.) But whatever its mechanism of action, acupuncture appears to work by balancing the movement of energy in the body.

Is acupuncture a simple process that can be performed by most anyone? *Absolutely not!* Acupuncturists spend many years mastering Oriental medical theory and learning the finesse required to combine points and perform acupuncture properly. As expert acupuncturist Giovanni Maciocia (1994) explained in his classic text, *The Practice of Chinese Medicine*:

> Combining points in a safe, effective, and harmonious way is a very important part of an acupuncture treatment. . . . Using points according to their action brings into play the particular nature of the individual point, while combining points in a harmonious way brings into play the channel system as a whole, and harmonizes Yin and Yang, Top and Bottom, Left and Right, and Front and Back. When points are combined well, the patient has an unmistakable feeling: it may be one of relaxation, elation, alertness, peacefulness or a combination of all these. Ideally, the patient should experience any of the above feelings during and after every treatment. (p. 805)

I can't emphasize strongly enough that Oriental medical theory is very complicated; it can't be learned in a weekend workshop. It takes many years to become proficient in all of the intricacies of tongue and pulse diagnosis, channel theory, organ theory, and point energetics. Interestingly, the licensing laws in many states currently allow licensed clinicians from other backgrounds (for example, medical doctors, naturopathic doctors, chiropractic doctors)—*with little or no training*—to practice TCM. This situation will perhaps change in the future as more and more people become licensed acupuncturists and build a stronger voice in state legislatures. In the meantime, I advise you to be careful when seeking a TCM practitioner. Only go to a licensed professional with adequate training in Oriental medicine. (See this chapter's Practical Pointer on selecting a complementary health practitioner.)

Clinical Applications of Acupuncture

Because acupuncture supports the body's natural healing powers, a majority of conditions can be improved, corrected, or even eliminated with TCM. This means the effectiveness of acupuncture extends far beyond the misconception that its only benefit is controlling pain. Acupuncture has repeatedly been shown to improve circulation, lower blood pressure, and increase the production of white and red blood cells. It can reduce gastric acidity and stimulate the immune system, as well as prompt the release of numerous hormones that assist the body's response to injury and stress.

According to data published by the World Health Organization (WHO), acupuncture is effective for eye and mouth disorders, respiratory and gastrointestinal disorders, and neurological and musculoskeletal disorders (Bannerman 1979). In the United States, acupuncture has historically been used to treat chronic pain conditions like headaches, arthritis, bursitis, injuries, and post-surgical pain. More recently, acupuncture has been used to treat mind-body problems like anxiety, stress, depression, insomnia, chronic fatigue, irritable bowel syndrome, hypertension, sexual dysfunctions, premenstrual symptoms, and menopausal symptoms. Some additional applications of acupuncture include treating drug and alcohol addictions, smoking, and eating disorders.

Acupuncture's efficacy for treating mind-body problems should be welcome news for sufferers of health anxiety syndrome.

The Healing Power of Plants: Chinese Herbs

Like acupuncture, Oriental herbal medicine is a comprehensive healing system that has been refined over thousands of years. It's also used worldwide. For instance, Japanese Kampo boasts an updated and proven approach to the ancient art of Oriental herbal medicine. In both the United States and Asian countries, the most common treatment protocol today involves combining Chinese herbs with acupuncture.

Regardless of the exact approach taken, Oriental herbal practitioners generally develop herbal prescriptions that are carefully tailored to each person's unique bodily constitution, primary symptoms, and chief complaints. In other words, the herbs are used holistically and not chosen based only on symptomatic complaints. This is quite a different approach than allopathic physicians take, which makes sense given the major philosophical differences between TCM and Western medicine.

According to Oriental medical theory, the human body is a composite of interacting component systems, with each part of the body influencing every other part of the body. TCM herbalists seek a complete description of every patient's overall health constitution and status in order to obtain precise results. In that way, the patient's unique patterns can be identified and the right herbal formula prescribed. Allopathic labels like influenza, arthritis, ulcer, hepatitis, allergies, heart disease, pneumonia, or premenstrual syndrome don't necessarily provide TCM herbalists with sufficient information.

The bottom line is that the use of Chinese herbs, like acupuncture, requires the expertise of a highly trained clinician. *Never use Chinese herbs except under the supervision of a qualified practitioner.*

Practical Pointer

Oriental herbs aren't "user-friendly" for novices. Because all of the body's component systems are intimately connected, to help you improve your health it's necessary to consider the entire complex of clinical signs and symptoms. In other words, all of your characteristics must be analyzed to determine the proper herbs for your unique situation. This requires an experienced TCM practitioner. You should also inform other health-care practitioners of any herbs you might be given to avoid potential adverse interactions with medications.

Oriental Medicine and Health Anxiety Syndrome

From the standpoint of TCM, anxiety is an emotion that is frequently associated with the "Organ systems" (the "Zang-Fu" energy systems) of the Liver and the Heart (although other energetic systems could be involved, too). While the notion of treating "Organ systems" probably sounds rather exotic and foreign to you, the idea is that generalized anxiety and fear can be reduced or eliminated using Oriental medicinal techniques.

As noted above, Oriental medicine is particularly effective for treating mind-body problems, including various forms of anxiety and psychosomatic illnesses. For example, an acupuncture point known as *Yin Tang*, which is located between the eyebrows, has a significant effect on most anxiety disturbances. And many Chinese herbal formulas for anxiety contain *Suan Zao Ren* (Semen Zizyphi Spinosae) because of its special calming properties.

In short, Chinese medicine offers an alternative explanation for how problems like health anxiety develop, as well as provides treatment techniques for dealing with your problems. Depending on your specific clinical presentation, acupuncture and herbal therapy could very well help in your recovery from health anxiety syndrome.

Practical Pointer

Selecting a qualified complementary health practitioner can be a daunting task. Following are a number of sample questions to consider asking as you screen potential health-care practitioners:

- *"Are you licensed by this state to practice?"*

- *"May I see your license to practice?"*

- *"What is your educational background and experience?"*

- *"How long have you been in practice?"*

- *"What is your predominant philosophy of healing?"*

- *"Do you have references I can contact?"*

- *"How do you arrive at a diagnosis?"*

- *"What does your treatment or therapy involve?"*

- *"What are the potential side effects of your treatment or therapy?"*

- *"What are the costs and duration of each treatment?"*

- *"Do you accept insurance? If so, which plans? If not, what kinds of financial arrangements are available?"*

- *"How long can I expect to be in treatment for my condition?"*

- *"How long can I expect to be in treatment before seeing results?"*

- *"Are you involved in any kind of teaching, ongoing research, and/or continuing education?"*

- *"Are you willing to consult with my other health-care practitioners, including medical doctors?"*

> - *"Do you mind if I share with my other health-care practitioners what treatments you recommend, so that I can avoid adverse interactions with the treatments I'm already receiving?"*
>
> Common sense suggests that you not proceed with treatment if your questions aren't answered to your satisfaction. You'll also want to avoid practitioners who:
>
> - *Criticize and negate all of allopathic medicine*
>
> - *Refuse to coordinate with other health-care professionals*
>
> - *Promise cures for incurable diseases*
>
> - *Want you to discontinue medications prescribed by your family doctor*
>
> - *Pressure you into purchasing expensive herbs, supplements, or devices*
>
> - *Require you to disrobe when your "gut" tells you it's inappropriate*
>
> - *Make you feel uncomfortable at any time*

Spirituality

Now that we've reviewed three popular models of alternative medicine, I'd also like to take a moment to mention *spiritual development* as an aid to overcoming health anxiety syndrome. As its own rather complex psychosocial concept, spirituality, or religious behavior and practice, is crucial to humanity's need to discover meaning in life. Spirituality—whether or not it involves active and formal membership in a religious organization—is an excellent tool for developing your desire and capacity for vision, purpose, and values attached to your existence. In other words, spirituality underlies ethics and morals, as well as the role that these play in the everyday actions that shape our lives.

Clearly, spirituality is important and satisfying to most of us, which explains why so many social scientists have taken a keen interest in this topic. It's been repeatedly found in research studies that spirituality and mental health are positively related, implying that the more spiritual you are, the more likely you'll have a healthy psyche and satisfying life.

So, ample evidence suggests that spiritual practices improve mental health in a variety of ways. Among its many benefits, regular spiritual practice can:

- Improve self-esteem and reduce anxiety and depression

- Contribute to helping people develop sound moral judgment and ethical principles

- Increase marital stability, happiness, and satisfaction

- Contribute to helping youth escape the perils of inner-city poverty, such as crime, delinquency, and substance abuse

- Inoculate people against various social problems, including divorce, suicide, alcohol and drug abuse, crime, and unintended pregnancies

- Reduce the likelihood of depression among young people experiencing the usual tensions of growing up in our modern world

- Reduce the likelihood of depression among those with medical conditions

- Enhance physical health—increasing longevity and lessening the incidence of serious diseases

- Improve the chances of recovery from illness

And how does all of this work? Besides God's role in our lives, researchers believe spirituality and religious practice positively influence the way we cognitively process life events. Restated simply, having a spiritual perspective helps you make sense of the world around you. And when you can do this, you're in a better position to rid yourself of your irrational thinking.

Conclusions

The field of mind-body psychology is moving closer and closer to a model of integration that combines the best therapies from a broad spectrum of Western and Eastern disciplines. Most complementary practices recognize the value of physical, mental, emotional, and spiritual aspects of wellness. Some therapies emphasize changing physical conditions through purely psychological interventions, while

For Personal Reflection

Emotions Anonymous is a twelve-step support group that is similar to Alcoholics Anonymous. Attendees suffer from such diverse problems as anxiety, panic, hypochondria, stress, tension, obsessions, compulsive behaviors, anger, depression, despair, social withdrawal, loneliness, grief, low self-esteem, jealousy, resentment, guilt, strained and broken relationships, exhaustion, indifference, negative thinking, and a host of other emotional issues.

Attendees meet at least weekly to process their emotions and learn effective coping strategies. Normally, this involves "working the twelve steps" of Emotions Anonymous with the help of a "sponsor" and group members.

The first three steps of Emotions Anonymous are:

1. We admitted we were powerless over our emotions—that our lives had become unmanageable.

2. Came to believe that a Power greater than ourselves could restore us to sanity.

3. Made a decision to turn our will and our lives over to the care of God as we understood Him.

How might these steps reflect the role of spirituality in overcoming emotional difficulties like health anxiety syndrome?

others emphasize changing these conditions through other means. Whatever their particular slant, these models hold that the human body is wonderfully resilient and—with some occasional coaxing and intervening—is capable of healing itself. This is why most holistic practitioners work with the entire person rather than treat symptoms and diseases. They also stress the importance of self-care and preventing sickness through a variety of means. The terms *complementary* and *integrative* reflect this unification of mind, body, and sprit.

While health anxiety syndrome presents a definite challenge to millions of Americans, healing is possible. And you've taken that all-important first step toward recovery by reading *Stop Worrying About Your Health!* May you find the life answers that you're looking for, as well as lasting freedom from whatever fears haunt you or your loved ones.

Feature: Healing Back Pain: John Sarno's Approach

The author of *Healing Back Pain: The Mind-Body Connection* is John Sarno (1994), an attending physician at the Rusk Institute of Rehabilitation Medicine, New York University Medical Center and a professor of Clinical Rehabilitation Medicine at New York University School of Medicine. Since the early 1970s, Dr. Sarno has conducted extensive research into pain syndromes, and has identified what he believes to be the cause of most neck, shoulder, limb, and back pain—something he refers to as *tension myositis syndrome* (TMS).

According to Sarno, TMS is a physically harmless condition typified by pain caused not by injuries or structural damage, but by a combination of daily life stresses and personality characteristics. It's his opinion that, once an actual physical cause of pain has been ruled out, you should look to the psyche as the culprit. He has explained it this way:

> The idea that pain means injury or damage is deeply ingrained in the American consciousness. Of course, if the pain starts while one is engaged in a physical activity it's difficult not to attribute the pain to the activity. (As we shall see later, that is often deceiving.) But this pervasive concept of the vulnerability of the back, of ease of injury, is nothing less than a medical catastrophe for the American public, which now has an army of semidisabled men and women whose lives are significantly restricted by the fear of doing further damage or bringing on the dreaded pain again. . . . The emotions do not lend themselves to test tube experiments and measurement and so modern medical science has chosen to ignore them, buttressed by the conviction that emotions have little to do with health and illness anyway. Hence, the majority of practicing physicians do not consider that emotions play a significant role in *causing* physical disorders, though many would acknowledge that they might aggravate a "physically" caused illness. In general, physicians feel uncomfortable in dealing with a

problem that is related to the emotions. They tend to make a sharp distinction between "the things of the mind" and "the things of the body," and only feel comfortable with the latter." (pp. 1–3)

Dr. Sarno's approach to the problem of pain is another example of the new medicine that recognizes the relationship between physical symptoms and emotions, as well as the power of cognitive processing to eliminate many common pain states.

Question for Thought: What do you think of John Sarno's assumption that most common pain syndromes are psychologically caused?

A Final Word

I hope you've enjoyed reading *Stop Worrying About Your Health!* and that you've gained at least a few new insights into the nature of your health worries, including strategies to overcome them. Although I can't promise to answer your letter, I'd like to hear from you concerning any impact that this book has had on your life. Feel free to contact me through my publisher.

Resources

Organizations

This section includes mental health, medical, and holistic health resources for sufferers of health anxiety syndrome, as well as their families and health-care providers:

Albert Ellis Institute (Institute for Rational-Emotive Therapy)
45 East 65th Street
New York, NY 10021
(800) 323-4738
www.REBT.org

American Academy of Child and Adolescent Psychiatry
3615 Wisconsin Avenue NW
Washington, DC 20016-3007
(202) 966-7300
www.aacap.org

American Counseling Association
5999 Stevenson Avenue
Alexandria, VA 22304
(703) 823-9800
www.counseling.org

American Chiropractic Association
1701 Clarendon Boulevard
Arlington, VA 22209
(800) 986-4636
www.amerchiro.org

American Institute for Cognitive Therapy
136 East 57th Street, Suite 1101
New York, NY 10022
(212) 308-2440
www.cognitivetherapynyc.com

American Massage Therapy Association
820 Davis Street
Evanston, IL 60201
(847) 864-0123
www.amtamassage.org

American Psychiatric Association
1400 K Street NW
Washington, DC 20005
(888) 357-7924
www.psych.org

American Psychological Association
750 First Street NE
Washington, DC 20002-4242
(800) 374-2721; (202) 336-5500
www.apa.org

Anxiety Disorders Association of America (ADAA)
11900 Parklawn Drive, Suite 100
Rockville, MD 20852
(301) 231-9350
www.adaa.org

Association for Advancement of Behavior Therapy (AABT)
305 Seventh Avenue, 16th Floor
New York, NY 10001-60008
(212) 647-1890
www.aabt.org

Council of Colleges of Acupuncture and Oriental Medicine
7501 Greenway Center Drive, Suite 820
Greenbelt, MD 20770

(301) 313-0868
www.ccaom.org

Emotions Anonymous International
P.O. Box 4245
St. Paul, MN 55104
(651) 647-9712
www.mtn.org/EA

International Paruresis Association
P.O. Box 26225
Baltimore, MD 21210
(800) 247-3864; (410) 938-8866
www.paruresis.org

International Society for Traumatic Stress Studies
60 Revere Drive, Suite 500
Northbrook, IL 60062
(847) 480-9028
www.istss.org

National Alliance for the Mentally Ill (NAMI)
Colonial Place Three, 2107 Wilson Boulevard, Suite 300
Arlington, VA 22201
(800) 950-NAMI
www.nami.org

National Association of Social Workers
750 First Street NE, Suite 700
Washington, DC 20002-4241
(800) 638-8799; (202) 408-8600
www.naswdc.org

National Institute of Mental Health
6001 Executive Boulevard, Room 8184, MSC 9663
Bethesda, MD 20892-9663
(800) 64-PANIC; (301) 443-4513
www.nimh.nih.gov

National Mental Health Association
1021 Prince Street
Alexandria, VA 22314-2971
(800) 969-NMHA; (703) 684-7722
www.nmha.org

For Further Reading

Below is a list of recommended readings (for both lay and professional readers) related to a variety of mind-body topics. For your convenience, I've divided the readings into a few broad categories:

Mind-Body Disorders, Health Psychology, Anxiety, Pain, and General Health

American Medical Association. 1995. *Diagnostic and Treatment Guidelines on Mental Health Effects of Family Violence*. Chicago, Ill: AMA.

American Psychiatric Association. 1994. *Diagnostic and Statistical Manual of Mental Disorders*, 4th ed. Washington, D.C.: AMA.

Anthony, M. M., and R. P. Swinson. 1998. *When Perfect Isn't Good Enough: Strategies for Coping with Perfectionism*. Oakland, Calif.: New Harbinger Publications.

Bakal, D. 1999. *Minding the Body: Clinical Uses of Somatic Awareness*. New York: Guilford Press.

Beck, A. T., G. Emery, and R. L. Greenberg. 1985. *Anxiety Disorders and Phobias*. New York: Basic Books.

Borysenko, J. 1988. *Minding the Body, Mending the Mind*. New York: Bantam.

Braiker, H. B. 1989. *The Type E Woman: How to Overcome the Stress of Being Everything to Everybody*. New York: NAL-Dutton.

Cameron, L., E. A. Leventhal, and H. Leventhal. 1995. Seeking medical care in response to symptoms and life stress. *Psychosomatic Medicine* 57:37-47.

Carey, B. 1996. The mind of a hypochondriac. *Health* 10(6):82.

Catalano, E. M. 1990. *Getting to Sleep*. Oakland, Calif.: New Harbinger Publications.

Catalano, E. M., and K. N. Hardin. 1996. *The Chronic Pain Control Workbook*. Oakland, Calif.: New Harbinger Publications.

Caudill, M. A. 1995. *Managing Pain Before It Manages You*. New York: Guilford Press.

Chaitow, L. 1990. *New Self-Help for Headaches and Migraine*. New York: HarperCollins.

Chaitow, L. 1993. *The Book of Pain Relief: A Comprehensive Self-Help Guide to Easing and Treating Both Chronic and Short-Term Pain*. San Francisco: Thorsons.

Cherniss, C. 1995. *Beyond Burnout: Helping Teachers, Nurses, Therapists, and Lawyers Recover from Stress and Disillusionment*. New York: Routledge.

Coren, S. 1996. *Sleep Thieves: An Eye-Opening Exploration into the Science and Mysteries of Sleep*. New York: The Free Press.

Damasio, A. R. 1994. *Descartes' Error: Emotion, Reason, and the Human Brain*. New York: G. P. Putnam's Sons.

Davis, M., E. R. Eshelman, and M. McKay. 1995. *The Relaxation and Stress Reduction Workbook*, 4th ed. Oakland, Calif.: New Harbinger Publications.

Dess, N. K. 2001. Frontiers: The new body-mind connection. *Psychology Today*, July/August, 30.

Donoghue, P., and M. Siegel. 1994. *Sick and Tired of Feeling Sick and Tired: Living with Invisible Chronic Illness*. New York: Norton Press.

Duckro, P. N., W. D. Richardson, and J. E. Marshall. 1995. *Taking Control of Your Headaches*. New York: Guilford.

Eimer, B. N., and A. Freeman. 1998. *Pain Management Psychother-apy: A Practical Guide*. New York: John Wiley & Sons.

Epstein, R. M., T. Quill, and I. R. McWhinney. 1999. Somatization reconsidered. *Archives of Internal Medicine* 159(3):215.

Fassel, D. 1993. *Working Ourselves to Death: And the Rewards of Recovery*. New York: HarperCollins.

Fink P. 1992. The use of hospitalizations by somatizing patients. *Psychological Medicine* 22:173–180.

Ford, C. V. 1983. *The Somatizing Disorders: Illness as a Way of Life*. New York: Elsevier Biomedical Press.

Freudenberger, H. J. 1980. *Burn-Out*. New York: Anchor Press.

Freudenberger, H. J., and G. North. 1990. *Women's Burnout: How to Spot It, How to Reverse It, How to Prevent It*. New York: Penguin Press.

Friedman, M., and R. H. Rosenman. 1974. *Type A Behavior and Your Heart*. New York: Alfred A. Knopf.

Griffith, J. L., and M. E. Griffith. 1994. *The Body Speaks: Therapeutic Dialogues for Mind-Body Problems*. New York: Basic Books.

Gureje, O., T. B. Ustun, and G. E. Simon. 1997. The syndrome of hypochondriasis: A cross-national study in primary care. *Psychological Medicine* 27:1001–1010.

Hafen, B. Q., K. J. Frandsen, K. J. Karren, and N. L. Smith. 1996. *Mind/Body Health: The Health Effects of Attitudes, Emotions, and Relationships*. Needham Heights, Mass.: Allyn and Bacon.

Hanson, R. W., and K. E. Gerber. 1989. *Coping with Chronic Pain: A Guide to Patient Self-Management*. New York: Guilford Press.

Hellman, C. J., M. Budd, J. Borysenko, D. C. McClelland, and H. Benson. 1990. A study of the effectiveness of two group behavioral medicine interventions for patients with psychosomatic complaints. *Behavioral Medicine* 16:165–173.

Johnson, S. L. 1997. *Therapist's Guide to Clinical Intervention: The 1-2-3s of Treatment Planning*. San Diego, Calif.: Academic Press.

Kaptchuk, T. J. 1983. *The Web That Has No Weaver: Understanding Chinese Medicine*. New York: Congdon & Weed.

Katon, W., E. Lin, M. Von Korff, J. Russo, F. Lipscomb, and T. Bush. 1991. Somatization: A spectrum of severity. *American Journal of Psychiatry* 148:34–40.

Keefe, F. J., J. Dunsmore, and R. Burnett. 1992. Behavioral and cognitive-behavioral approaches to chronic pain: Recent advances and future directions. *Journal of Consulting and Clinical Psychology* 60:528–536.

Kellner, R. 1991. *Psychosomatic Syndromes and Somatic Symptoms*. Washington, D.C.: American Psychiatric Press.

Kirmayer, L. I., and J. M. Robbins. 1996. Patients who somatize in primary care: A longitudinal study of cognitive and social characteristics. *Psychological Medicine* 26:937–951.

Kleinman, A. 1988. *The Illness Narratives*. New York: HarperCollins.

Lark, S. 1989. *PMS: Premenstrual Syndrome Self-Help Book*. Berkeley, Calif.: Celestial Arts.

Leff, G. P. 1988. *Psychiatry Around the Globe: A Transcultural View*, 2nd ed. London: Gaskell.

Lipowski, Z. J. 1988. Somatization: The concept and its clinical application. *American Journal of Psychiatry* 145:1358–1368.

Lorig, K., H. Holman, D. Sobel, et al. 1994. *Living a Healthy Life with Chronic Conditions: Self-Management of Heart Disease, Arthritis, Stroke, Diabetes, Asthma, Bronchitis, Emphysema and Others*. Menlo Park, Calif.: Bull Publishing.

Mallinger, A. E., and J. DeWyze. 1992. *Too Perfect: When Being in Control Gets Out of Control*. New York: Clarkson Potter Publishers.

Martin, P. R. 1993. *Psychological Management of Chronic Headaches*. New York: Guilford.

Mayou, R., C. Bass, and M. Sharpe, eds. 1995. *Treatment of Functional Somatic Symptoms*. New York: Oxford University Press.

Melzack, R., and P. D. Wall. 1982. *The Challenge of Pain*. New York: Penguin.

Moyers, B. 1992. *Healing and the Mind*. New York: Doubleday.

Ornstein, R., and D. Sobel. 1989. *Healthy Pleasures*. New York: Addison-Wesley.

Ornstein, R., and C. Swencionis, eds. 1990. *The Healing Brain: A Scientific Reader*. New York: Guilford Press.

Othmer, E. 1994. *The Clinical Interview Using DSM-IV*. Washington, D.C.: American Psychiatric Press.

Papalia, D. E., and S. W. Olds. 1995. *Human Development*, 6th ed. New York: McGraw-Hill.

Pennebaker, J. W. 1982. *The Psychology of Physical Symptoms*. New York: Springer-Verlag.

———. 1997. *Opening Up: The Healing Power of Expressing Emotions*. New York: Guilford Press.

Perl, J. 1993. *Sleep Right in Five Nights*. New York: Morrow.

Peveler, R., L. Kilkenny, and A. L. Kinmonth. 1997. Medically unexplained physical symptoms in primary care: A comparison of self-report screening questionnaires and clinical opinion. *Journal of Psychosomatic Research* 42:245-52.

Rolland, J. S. 1994. *Families, Illness and Disability: An Integrative Treatment Model*. New York: Basic Books.

Sarno, J. 1994. *Healing Back Pain*. New York: Warner Books.

Smith, M. J. 1975. *When I Say No, I Feel Guilty*. New York: Bantam Books.

Soifer, S., G. D. Zgourides, J. Himle, and N. L. Pickering. 2001. *Shy Bladder Syndrome: Your Step-By-Step Guide to Overcoming Paruresis*. Oakland, Calif.: New Harbinger Publications.

Stewart, M., J. B. Brown, W. W. Weston, I. R. McWhinney, C. L. McWilliam, and T. R. Freeman. 1995. *Patient-Centered Medicine: Transforming the Clinical Method*. Thousand Oaks, Calif.: Sage Publications.

Swedo, S., and H. Leonard. 1996. *It's Not All in Your Head: Now Women Can Discover the Real Causes of Their Most Commonly Misdiagnosed Health Problems*. San Francisco: HarperCollins.

Temoshok, L. 1992. *The Type C Connection*. New York: Random House.

U.S. Department of Health and Human Services (USDHHS). 2000. *Healthy People 2010* (Conference Edition, in two volumes). Washington, D.C.: USDHHS.

Ustun, T. B., N. Sartorius, eds. 1995. *Mental Illness in General Health Care: An International Study*. New York: John Wiley & Sons.

Varela, F. J., E. Thompson, and E. Rosch. 1991. *The Embodied Mind: Cognitive Science and Human Experience*. Cambridge, Mass.: MIT Press.

Wall, P. D., and R. Melzack. 1984. *Textbook of Pain*. New York: Churchill Livingstone.

Warren, R., and G. D. Zgourides. 1991. *Anxiety Disorders: A Rational-Emotive Perspective.* Needham Heights, Mass.: Allyn and Bacon.

Williams, R. 1989. *The Trusting Heart.* New York: Times Books.

Zgourides, G. 1996. *Human Sexuality: Contemporary Perspectives.* New York: HarperCollins.

———. 2000. *Developmental Psychology.* Foster City, Calif.: IDG Books.

Imagery, Visualization, Desensitization, Hypnosis, Relaxation, and Rational-Emotive Behavior Therapy

Baker, R. A. 1990. *They Call It Hypnosis.* Buffalo, N.Y.: Prometheus.

Benson, H. 1992. *The Relaxation Response.* New York: Wing Books.

Berkow, R., ed. 1992. *The Merck Manual of Diagnosis and Therapy,* 16th ed. Rahway, N.J.: Merck Research Laboratories.

Berne, E. 1964. *Games People Play.* New York: Grove Press.

Bowers, K. S. 1983. *Hypnosis: For the Seriously Curious.* New York: Norton.

Brown, D. P., and E. Fromm. 1987. *Hypnosis and Behavioral Medicine.* Hillsdale, N.J.: Erlbaum.

Burns, D. D. 1980. *Feeling Good: The New Mood Therapy.* New York: William Morrow.

———. 1989. *The Feeling Good Handbook.* New York: William Morrow.

Cantor, C., and B. Fallon. 1996. *Phantom Illness: Recognizing, Understanding, and Overcoming Hypochondria.* Boston: Mariner.

Clarke, J. C., and J. A. Jackson. 1983. *Hypnosis and Behavior Therapy: The Treatment of Anxiety and Phobias.* New York: Springer.

Crabtree, A. 1988. *Animal Magnetism, Early Hypnotism, and Psychical Research, 1766-1925: An Annotated Bibliography.* Millwood, N.Y.: Kraus.

Crasilneck, H. B., and J. A. Hall. 1985. *Clinical Hypnosis: Principles and Applications.* Orlando, Fla.: Grune & Stratton.

Dempcy, M. H., and R. Tihista. 1996. *Dear Job Stressed: Answers for the Overworked, Overwrought, and Overwhelmed*. Palo Alto, Calif.: Davies-Black Publishing.

Eagley, A. H., and S. Chaiken. 1993. *The Psychology of Attitudes*. Fort Worth, Tex.: Harcourt Brace Jovanovich.

Edmonston, W. E. 1986. *The Induction of Hypnosis*. New York: Wiley.

Ellis, A. 1957. *How to Live with a Neurotic*. New York: Crown Publishers.

———. 1962. *Reason and Emotion in Psychotherapy*. New York: Lyle Stuart.

———. 1965, 1994. Showing people they are not worthless individuals. *Voices: The Art and Science of Psychotherapy* 1(2):74–77 (Revised, 1994).

———. 1971. *Growth Through Reason*. Palo Alto, Calif.: Science and Behavior Books.

———. 1986. Anxiety about anxiety: The use of hypnosis with rational-emotive therapy. In *Case Studies in Hypnotherapy*, edited by E. T. Dowd and J. M. Healy. New York: Guilford Press.

———. 1988. *How to Stubbornly Refuse to Make Yourself Miserable About Anything—Yes, Anything!* Secaucus, N.J.: Lyle & Stuart.

———. 1993. Rational-emotive imagery and hypnosis. In *Handbook of Clinical Hypnosis*, edited by J. W. Rhue, S. J. Lynn, and I. Kirsch. Washington, D.C.: American Psychological Association.

———. 1999. *How to Make Yourself Happy and Remarkably Less Disturbable*. San Luis Obispo, Calif.: Impact Publishers.

Ellis, A., and M. E. Bernard, eds. 1985. *Clinical Applications of Rational-Emotive Therapy*. New York: Plenum.

Ellis, A., and W. Dryden. 1987. *The Practice of Rational-Emotive Therapy*. New York: Springer.

Ellis, A., J. Gordon, M. Neenan, and S. Palmer. 1997. *Stress Counseling: A Rational-Emotive Behavior Approach*. London: Cassell.

Ellis, A., and R. Grieger, eds. *Handbook of Rational-Emotive Therapy* (2 vols.). New York: Springer.

Ellis, A., and R. A. Harper. 1975. *A New Guide to Rational Living*. Hollywood: Wilshire Books.

Erickson, M. H. 1982. *My Voice Will Go with You: The Teaching Tales of Milton H. Erickson.* New York: Norton.

Evangelista, A. 1991. *Dictionary of Hypnosis.* Westport, Conn.: Greenwood.

Fromm, E., and S. Kahn. 1990. *Self-Hypnosis: The Chicago Paradigm.* New York: Guilford Press.

Hall, J. A. 1990. *Hypnosis: A Jungian Perspective.* New York: Guilford Press.

Hammond, D. C., ed. 1990. *Handbook of Hypnotic Suggestions and Metaphors.* New York: W. W. Norton & Company.

Heap, M. 1988. *Hypnosis: Current Clinical, Experimental, and Forensic Practices.* New York: Routledge.

Lazarus, A. A. 1984. *In the Mind's Eye.* New York: Guilford Press.

Lazarus, A. A., and C. N. Lazarus. 1998. *The 60-Second Shrink: 101 Strategies for Staying Sane in a Crazy World.* San Luis Obispo, Calif.: Impact Publishers.

Lazarus, A. A., C. N. Lazarus, and A. Fay. 1993. *Don't Believe It for a Minute: Forty Toxic Ideas That Are Driving You Crazy.* San Luis Obispo, Calif.: Impact Publishers.

Loftus, E. F., and K. Ketcham. 1994. *The Myth of Repressed Memory: False Memories and Allegations of Sexual Abuse.* New York: St. Martin's Press.

Maltz, M. 1960. *Psycho-Cybernetics.* New York: Pocket Books.

McKay, M., and P. Fanning. 2000. *Self-Esteem,* 3rd ed. Oakland, Calif.: New Harbinger Publications.

Naish, P. L. N. 1987. *What Is Hypnosis? Current Theories and Research.* New York: Taylor & Francis.

Oughourlian, J.-M. 1991. *The Puppet of Desire: The Psychology of Hysteria, Possession, and Hypnosis.* Stanford, Calif.: Stanford University Press.

Palmer, S., and W. Dryden. 1995. *Counseling for Stress Problems.* London: Sage.

Palmer, S., W. Dryden, A. Ellis, and R. Yapp, eds. 1995. *Rational Interviews.* London: Centre for Rational Emotive Behavior Therapy.

Pierce, W. D., and W. F. Epling, 1995. *Behavior Analysis and Learning.* New Jersey: Prentice-Hall, Inc.

Rhue, J. W., S. J. Lynn, I. Kirsch, eds. 1993. *Handbook of Clinical Hypnosis*. Washington, D.C.: American Psychological Association.

Sanders, S. 1990. *Clinical Self-Hypnosis*. New York: Guilford Press.

Scheflin, A. W., and J. L. Shapiro. 1990. *Trance on Trial*. New York: Guilford Press.

Schoenberger, N. E. 1996. Cognitive-behavioral hypnotherapy for phobic anxiety. In *Casebook of Clinical Hypnosis*, edited by S. J. Lynn, I. Kirsch, and J. W. Rhue. Washington, D.C.: American Psychological Association.

Spanos, N. P., and J. F. Chaves, eds. 1988. *Hypnosis: The Cognitive-Behavioral Perspective*. Buffalo, N.Y.: Prometheus.

Torrey, E. F. 1992. *Freudian Fraud: The Malignant Effect of Freud's Theory on American Thought and Culture*. New York: Harper-Collins.

Tosi, D. J., and M. A. Murphy. 1994. Cognitive hypnotherapy in psychosomatic illness: A cognitive experiential perspective. *Journal of Cognitive Psychotherapy: An International Quarterly* 8:4.

Udolf, R. 1987. *Handbook of Hypnosis for Professionals*. New York: Van Nostrand Reinhold.

Zilbergeld, B., M. G. Edelstein, and D. L. Araoz. 1986. *Hypnosis: Questions and Answers*. New York: Norton.

Spirituality and Mental Health

Bergin, A. E. 1991. Values and religious issues in psychotherapy and mental health. *American Psychologist* 46(4):394.

Bergin, A. E., K. S. Masters, and P. S. Richards. 1987. Religiousness and mental health reconsidered: A study of an intrinsically religious sample. *Journal of Counseling Psychology* 34(2):197.

Bergin, A. E., R. D. Stinchfield, T. A. Gaskin, K. S. Masters, and C. E. Sullivan. 1988. Religious life-styles and mental health: An exploratory study. *Journal of Counseling Psychology* 35(1):91.

Hunsberger, B. 1985. Religion, age, life satisfaction, and perceived sources of religiousness: A study of older persons. *Journal of Gerontology* 40(5):615–620.

Jensen, L. C., J. Jensen, and T. Wiederhold. 1993. Religiosity, denomination, and mental health among young men and women. *Psychological Reports* 72(3, Pt 2):1157–1158.

Kroll, J. 1995. Religion and psychiatry. *Current Opinion in Psychiatry* 8:335-339.

Levin, J. S., and H. Y. Vanderpool. 1987. Is frequent religious attendance really conducive to better health? Toward an epidemiology of religion. *Social Science and Medicine* 24(7):589–600.

Spilka, B., and D. N. McIntosh, eds. 1996. *The Psychology of Religion: Theoretical Approaches.* Boulder, Colo.: Westview.

References

American Psychiatric Association. 2000. *Diagnostic and Statistical Manual of Mental Disorders*, 4th ed., text rev. Washington, D.C.: APA.

Antony, M. M., and R. P. Swinson. 1998. *When Perfect Isn't Good Enough: Strategies for Coping with Perfectionism*. Oakland, Calif.: New Harbinger Publications.

Balch, J. F., and P. A. Balch. 1997. *Prescription for Nutritional Healing*, 2nd ed. New York: Avery.

Bannerman, R. H. 1979. Acupuncture: the WHO view. *World Health, December*, 27–28.

Beck, A. T., G. Emery, and R. L. Greenberg. 1985. *Anxiety Disorders and Phobias*. New York: Basic Books.

Burns, D. D. 1989. *The Feeling Good Handbook*. New York: William Morrow.

Cantor, C., and B. Fallon. 1996. *Phantom Illness: Recognizing, Understanding, and Overcoming Hypochondria*. Boston: Mariner.

Carmelli, D., A. Dame, G. Swan, and R. Rosenman 1991. Long-term changes in Type A behavior: a 27-year follow-up of the Western Collaborative Group Study. *Journal of Behavioral Medicine* 14:593–606.

Castleman, M. 2000. *Blended Medicine: The Best Choices in Healing.* New York: Rodale.

Cherkin, D. C., D. Eisenberg, K. J. Sherman, et al. 2001. Randomized trial comparing traditional Chinese medical acupuncture, therapeutic massage, and self-care education for chronic low back pain. *Archives of Internal Medicine* 161:1081–1088.

Coelho, L. R. 1997. *Applied Chiropractic.* Fort Worth, Tex.: Share International II.

Davis, M., E. R. Eshelman, and M. McKay. 2000. *The Relaxation and Stress Reduction Workbook,* 5th ed. Oakland, Calif.: New Harbinger Publications.

Ellis, A. 1962. *Reason and Emotion in Psychotherapy.* New York: Lyle Stuart.

———. 1982. Psychoneurosis and anxiety problems. In *Cognitive and Emotional Disturbance,* edited by R. Grieger and I. Grieger. New York: Human Sciences Press.

———. 1988. *How to Stubbornly Refuse to Make Yourself Miserable About Anything—Yes, Anything!* Secaucus, N.J.: Lyle & Stuart.

Johnson, S. L. 1997. *Therapist's Guide to Clinical Intervention: The 1-2-3s of Treatment Planning.* San Diego, Calif.: Academic Press.

Lazarus, A. A., and C. N. Lazarus. 1997. *The 60-Second Shrink: 101 Strategies for Staying Sane in a Crazy World.* San Luis Obispo, Calif.: Impact Publishers.

Lazarus, A. A., C. N. Lazarus, and A. Fay. 1993. *Don't Believe It for a Minute! Forty Toxic Ideas That Are Driving You Crazy.* San Luis Obispo, Calif.: Impact Publishers.

Kellner, R. 1991. *Psychosomatic Syndromes and Somatic Symptoms.* Washington, D.C.: American Psychiatric Press.

Maciocia, G. 1994. *The Practice of Chinese Medicine: The Treatment of Diseases with Acupuncture and Chinese Herbs.* London: Churchill Livingstone.

Mallinger, A. E., and J. DeWyze. 1992. *Too Perfect: When Being in Control Gets Out of Control.* New York: Clarkson Potter Publishers.

Mann, F. 1973. *Acupuncture: The Ancient Chinese Art of Healing and How It Works Scientifically.* New York: Vintage Books.

Rosenman, R. H., and M. Friedman. 1963. Behavior patterns, blood lipids, and coronary heart disease. *Journal of the American Medical Association* 184:934.

Sarno, J. E. 1991. *Healing Back Pain: The Mind-Body Connection.* New York: Warner Books.

Selye, H. 1976. *The Stress of Life.* New York: McGraw-Hill.

Soifer, S., G. D. Zgourides, J. Himle, and N. L. Pickering. 2001. *Shy Bladder Syndrome: Your Step-By-Step Guide to Overcoming Paruresis.* Oakland, Calif.: New Harbinger Publications.

Tappan, F. M. 1988. *Healing Massage Techniques: Holistic, Classic, and Emerging Methods,* 2nd ed. East Norwalk, Conn.: Appleton & Lange.

Wolpe, J. 1958. *Psychotherapy by Reciprocal Inhibition.* Stanford: Stanford University Press.

Lightning Source UK Ltd.
Milton Keynes UK
13 May 2010

154127UK00002B/120/P